Your Inner Engine:
An Introductory Course on Human Metabolism

Jane M. Vanderkooi
University of Pennsylvania

Forward

I began writing this book when I was starting chemotherapy. As the chemo treatment advanced, I was curious about how the drugs were exactly working. I wondered whether it would be possible for someone without a science background to get an understanding of human metabolism. I am attempting here to give an explanation of metabolism.

In this book, the few chemical formulae that are given are explained. I do not assume that you already have a background in organic chemistry, but if you do, the chemical formulae given can be a review for you. This book will be useful for someone to study before starting a more detailed Biochemistry course, since here an overview is given. It is written for the general public, but especially for people who are in health care. Each chapter begins with an overview. If you have never studied biochemistry, you can consider reading these overviews (1.1, 2.1, 3.1...) first, and then go back to examine the whole book.

There is a bit to learn. You can know what "bon jour" and "merci bien" mean in French, but you need a bigger vocabulary and understanding of grammar before you can understand written and spoken French. The same is true in metabolism. Some one may give advice (say, "Eat blueberries; they are high in anti-oxidants"), but to evaluate whether the advice is good, you must have a general over-all knowledge of metabolism.

I would like to thank my colleagues at the University of Pennsylvania for many years of friendship and intellectual stimulation. I also thank my family members for their help and many friends who made constructive comments on the book. I thank the students of Ann Minnick's class at Northwestern College, Orange City Iowa, for their constructive criticism and help with this book.

Your Inner Engine:

An Introductory Course on Human Metabolism

JANE M VANDERKOOI, Ph.D.

Contents

1. An inner engine keeps us alive

For an engine to run, it needs fuel. To live, we also need fuel. In the animal kingdom, fuel is provided by the breakdown of foods. Hence, in order to stay alive, grow and perform many necessary functions, we, the humans, require constant supply of foodstuff. The breakdown of food and conversion to energy is called metabolism. The word comes from Greek *meta* and *ballein*, meaning "to throw". So, "metabolism" refers to chemical changes that "throw into a different position", or covert food into energy in living tissues.

Let us illustrate the need of fuel in the living brain. Brain, like all the other body's organs, has its own peculiar food requirement. Unlike some organs, the brain is active at all times.

The key metabolic fuels, i.e. molecules whose combustion produces energy, are carbohydrates (sugar is a carbohydrate), proteins and fats. Under a usual eating schedule, when breakfast, lunch and dinner is eaten, brain relies almost exclusively on sugar and only during long-term starvation does it indirectly switch to fat for fuel.

The story of the gingerbread person (GB) shows what happens to brain metabolism after eating and during fasting.

It is 3 P.M. and GB eats a big piece of cake at a birthday party. Sugar from the cake goes into the digestive tract, where it is modified, and from there, into the blood. Circulating blood delivers the sugar to the brain, which uses sugar to generate energy to stay alive and to function.

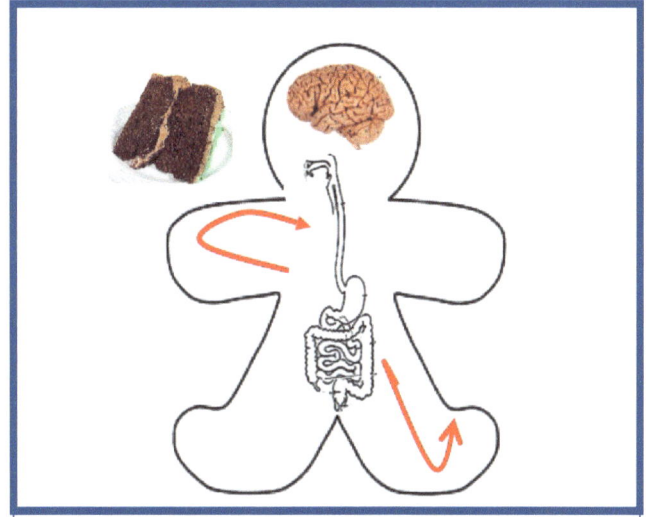

Figure 1.1. GB eats a big piece of cake. Sugar goes into intestine and then to circulating blood. This sugar is used as fuel for the brain.

After the party GB works hard on school assignments and does not eat for several hours. The sugar *from the cake* is no longer in his bloodstream, yet GB's brain appears to function perfectly well! How is it possible? Where does the fuel come from? It comes from a storage form of glucose (a sugar) called glycogen, which was produced in the liver from sugar present in the birthday cake. Breakdown of glycogen liberates glucose, which is delivered to brain through the circulation of blood.

GB goes skateboarding for two hours, and then he slowly walks home. GB's brain remains functioning even though his muscles are also using fuel.

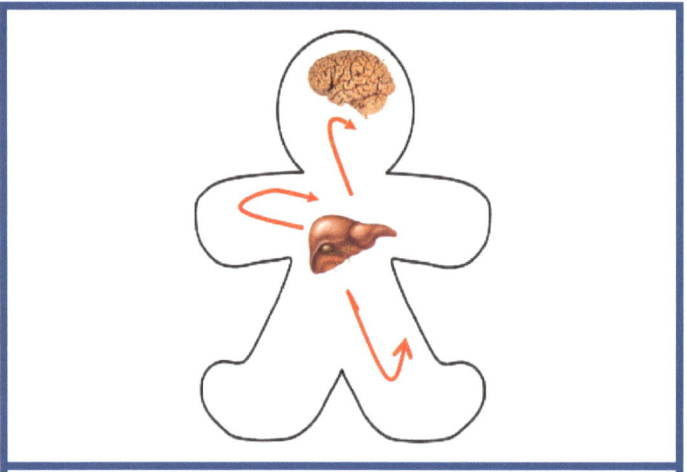

Figure 1.2. GB has not eaten for several hours. Glycogen from liver is released into blood as glucose, and the brain uses the circulating glucose for energy.

GB is now tired and goes to bed without eating. He wakes up in the morning hungry but refreshed and perfectly fine. His brain was not idle even for a moment during the night and, hence, continually needed fuel. Where did glucose come from this time? After exhaustion of liver glycogen (which takes 6-8 hrs) glucose was made in the liver using amino acids that were taken from muscle and other proteins. (Several other small molecules were made into glucose too). Released into the circulation from liver, glucose was eventually taken into brain and used for energy to support its functions.

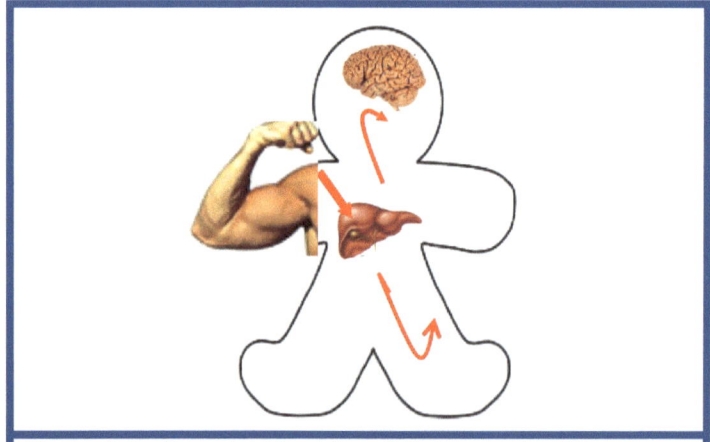

Figure 1.3. Overnight fast, i.e., GB does not eat for more than about eight to 12 hours. Glucose is still circulating in blood, but this glucose does not come from ingested glucose. Instead, muscle proteins are broken down, and liver makes glucose from them. This glucose goes into circulation and is used by brain.

Many years later, GB can not eat. This may be because GB develops a disease which prevents him from eating, or there is a famine and food is not available. Consequently, there are no sources of sugar in the digestive tract. After a couple of days stored glycogen has also been exhausted and glucose in GB's blood has fallen. Yet, GB is still able to think clearly; what is the metabolic fuel for his brain?

Under such condition, called "starvation", brain defends itself from death by switching to the use fat that is stored in the adipose tissue. Fat travels to the liver via circulation where it is converted to compounds called ketoacids. The latter are released from the liver and delivered via blood stream to the brain. GB is getting thinner and thinner as his fat is being used up.

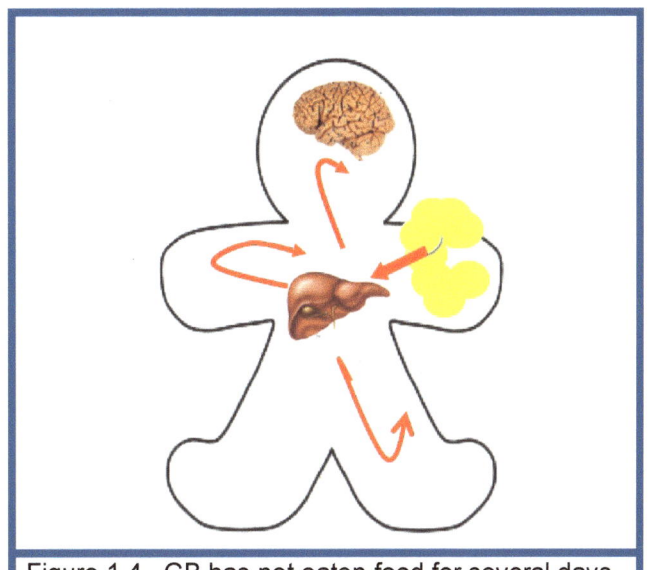

Figure 1.4. GB has not eaten food for several days. Fat is broken down. Liver converts fat into ketoacids. The brain's metabolism changes so that it can use ketoacids for energy.

Under extreme starvation, muscle proteins continue to be gradually broken up and amino acids from these proteins are used for the synthesis of glucose. Without food, eventually, heart and diaphragm muscles can no longer function.

Why does brain use mostly sugar for energy? Why does it not also use fat, like most other tissues? No one knows the answer to this, but our focus on the brain shows how intriguing metabolism is. Brain relies on the stomach and intestine for sugar after eating. For intermediate times, a store of glycogen in liver supplies glucose. Later, liver uses amino acids from protein to make new glucose for the brain. During long starvation, fat is broken down, and the liver makes ketoacids that are used for fuel in the nervous system.

At all times, whether feasting or fasting, GB's blood carries oxygen and metabolic fuels while organs of his body perform their many duties and functions. GB's brain uses 120 g of glucose per day whether GB is exercising, thinking hard or not thinking about much and receives 20% of blood supply. This is about 500 calories. During one day, the heart pumps about 8 ton of blood. Whereas the brain uses glucose for energy, the heart is using mostly fat as an energy source. In humans, metabolism of fat requires oxygen, and at all times GB is breathing and obtaining oxygen through the lungs. Waste materials are always being formed and are eliminated by the kidney into the urine (metabolic by-products) and into the atmosphere by the lungs (carbon dioxide).

The metabolism of one organ depends upon the metabolism of other organs. All must be functioning to ensure health and wellbeing. The inner engine shows a marvelously complex and balanced interdependence of parts.

2. Nuts and bolts of the machine: Atoms and molecules of life

2.1 We are composed mostly of oxygen, carbon, hydrogen and nitrogen

A Google search reveals that a car has about 14,000 parts. A fighter plane has about 240,000 parts. When you open the hood of the car, the complexity of the engine may startle you. But, the principles of construction are not that complicated. For instance, to attach two sheets of metal together, you use a bolt. To stabilize the bolt so that it does not fall out, a nut is needed. There are hundreds of thousands different molecules in the body, built from atoms. Atoms form molecules by combining in certain rules, just as nuts and bolts are always connected. You do not need to know all the molecules of the body, but you must have some understanding of most of them are built and how they work.

We are composed of only a few types of atoms. The "nut and bolts" of our molecules are predominately only four atom types: oxygen (O), carbon (C), hydrogen (H) and nitrogen (N). There are a few more atom types that we will introduce later, but if you know how these four atoms combine into molecules, you can understand how more complicated molecules are formed and act. In organic chemistry there are thousands of molecules that can be made from these four atoms. Fortunately, we can simplify our task by considering big, complex molecules as being composed of smaller, simpler ones.

The simple molecules are water (H_2O), carbon dioxide (CO_2), oxygen gas (O_2) and ammonia (NH_3).

2.2 Simple molecules

You learned in grade school that H_2O is the chemical formula water. Water is composed of hydrogen, H, and oxygen, O. The subscript means that each water molecule has two H atoms. When there is no subscript, it means that there is one atom. Thus a water molecule has one O. We need water to digest our food, transport our nutrients through the blood and regulate temperature. Our bodies also make H_2O. When we metabolize food, water is formed.

There is more than one way to write H_2O. Other ways are:

HOH or H-O-H

A dash indicates that one atom is attached to another. In other words, in H-O-H there is a bond from one H to O, and a bond from the other H to O. Here are two rules (equivalent to rules of grammar):

   1. Oxygen can form a bond with two other atoms; you see that in H_2O, O has one bond each with the two H's.
   2. H can form a bond with one other atom.

We are composed mostly of water. About 75 to 80% of a newborn baby is water. As we age, our body content decreases and the water content of an elderly person can be about 50-70% water. (With age, we shrink like a raisin!). We humans need more water than many other species, but it appears that all life on earth requires water.

The next important molecule that we need to know about is oxygen. Oxygen that we breathe from the atmosphere is the gaseous molecule O_2. Molecular oxygen is composed of two oxygen atoms, as you can tell from the subscript. Another way to write O_2 is:

$$O=O$$

You see that each O atom forms two bonds with the other O molecule. This is how it fulfills the rule that O has two bonds. The word "oxygen" is used to describe both the molecule O_2 and the atom. When we say that sugars contain oxygen, we mean that they contain the element O.

Another simple molecule is CO_2. It is called carbon dioxide. It is composed of one carbon atom and two oxygen atoms. Another way to write CO_2 is

$$O=C=O$$

Carbon atoms can form four bonds. In carbon dioxide, C forms two bonds with each oxygen atom.

With these compounds we can state what occurs in metabolism. The over all process is:

Food (containing carbon, hydrogen, oxygen) + O_2 (from air) → CO_2 and H_2O

The reaction written above says that our food combines with oxygen to form carbon dioxide and water. This process provides all the energy for our body.

Oxygen, O_2, comes from the atmosphere and we get it from **breathing**. Carbon, hydrogen and oxygen come from the food that we **eat**. This reaction, food combining with O_2, must be going on at all times. Human do not store much O_2, hence if we stop breathing, our brain is not getting O_2 and the above reaction cannot give energy to the brain. Without O_2 we will die quickly, within minutes. Without food we will also die, but we store food in our body, so that we do not have to be eating all the time. If we are "pleasantly plump" we can live for several days, weeks or even months on the fat stored in our bodies.

The food that we eat, -- carbohydrates (sugars and starches, composed of H, O and C) and fats (composed mainly of C and H) -- react with O_2 to form CO_2 and H_2O. No atoms disappear during metabolism. When we lose weight, we are breathing out CO_2, which goes to the atmosphere. The C's lost as CO_2 had been stored in our body as fat.

Our food also includes proteins. Proteins contain C, O and H, and these are metabolized to form CO_2 and H_2O, the end products of metabolism of fat and carbohydrate. But proteins also contain another element, nitrogen, N. To talk about N, the small molecule that we introduce is ammonia. Ammonia is:

$$NH_3.$$

Another way to write ammonia is:

$$H-\underset{\underset{H}{|}}{\overset{N}{\diagdown}}H$$

Ammonia is a pyramidal-shaped molecule; this is why the H's are drawn in a skewed way in the second drawing. CO_2 and H_2O are planar as they have only three atoms (you may remember from geometry that three points define a plane). Ammonia is a gas, but when it is in water it takes an H atom from a water molecule and it becomes NH_4^+, the ammonium ion:

$$H-\underset{\underset{H}{|}}{\overset{\overset{H}{|}}{N}}{}^{+}H$$

It now has a positive charge. Ammonium ion is not a gas. We use solutions of ammonium to clean windows, and some of the ammonium ions, NH_4^+, in the water escape the water and become ammonia, NH_3. Ammonia gas is very smelly and toxic.

Nitrogen is essential because we need proteins in our bodies. Proteins do many things; for instance, hemoglobin that makes blood red is a protein. Its function is to transport oxygen to the tissues of our body. Proteins make up molecules called enzymes. Enzymes determine what kind of chemical reactions occur our body. Nitrogen is also found in nucleic acids that form DNA. DNA makes up our genetic material and DNA determines the structure of all of the proteins in our bodies.

We need to eat protein to obtain N. Although, nitrogen is essential to life, we also have to get rid of excess nitrogen. The ultimate product of N as a by-product of protein metabolism is NH_3. Some fish species get rid of N by excreting NH_3. Our bodies do not do this, which is fortunate because NH_3 is so toxic – and besides we would not be popular with our fellow humans if a smelly, obnoxious cloud of ammonia surrounded us at all times! Our body gets rid of NH_3 by forming urea. This is urea:

$$H_2N-\overset{\overset{O}{\|}}{C}-NH_2$$

Ammonia and CO_2 combine to make urea as follows:

$$2NH_3 + CO_2 \rightarrow H_2N-\overset{\overset{O}{\|}}{C}-NH_2 + H_2O$$

This reaction states that two ammonia molecules, NH_3, combine with one CO_2 molecule to form urea. Unlike ammonia, urea is not toxic nor is particularly smelly. For humans, urea is the end-product of the metabolism of proteins. It dissolves in water and it is excreted from the body in urine.

In summary, the final products of metabolism are H_2O, CO_2 and NH_3 (excreted as urea). The important small molecules are listed in Table 1.

Table 1. Small molecules of metabolism

Name	Formula	Where they come from or where they go
oxygen	O_2	Obtained from breathing air
water	H_2O or HOH	Product of metabolism
carbon dioxide	CO_2 or O=C=O	Product of metabolism, excreted by breathing
ammonia	NH_3	Product of protein metabolism
urea	NH_2CONH_2.	Made from CO_2 and NH_3. Excreted in urine.

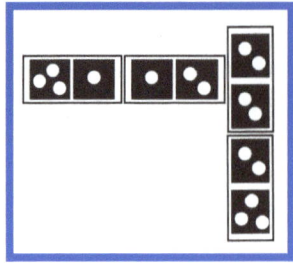

2.3 Complex molecules of food can be considered in terms of 1, 2 and 3 C's

Foods that we eat are much more complicated than the simple molecules that are the products of metabolism. All food molecules contain carbon, C. The subspecialty of chemistry that deals with carbon molecules is called organic chemistry.[1] Organic chemistry is a vast field. Just as there are many ways to combine dominos, there are many ways to arrange C in molecules.

Most courses in biochemistry require the student to take one year of organic chemistry before studying biochemistry. Although there are many organic compounds, a big simplification is to consider whether the compounds are made up of one C, two C or three C units. Just as in dominos, there are still many possible combinations, but large molecules will not daunt us when we think of them as composed of small units

To explain this, the first organic molecules that we consider are methane, ethane, and propane:

$$methane, CH_4$$
$$ethane, C_2H_6$$
$$propane, C_3H_8$$

A small amount of methane is produced in our intestinal tract by bacteria. We ourselves do not produce CH_4, C_2H_6 and C_3H_8 and we do not eat these compounds. Methane, CH_4, is the primary component of natural gas – surely not an appetizing meal! But these compounds are important because they form the basis of other molecules.

Methane can also be written as follows (the second structure is drawn to show that it is three-dimensional):

$$H-\overset{\displaystyle H}{\underset{\displaystyle H}{C}}-H \qquad \overset{\displaystyle H}{\underset{H\quad H}{C}}$$

Ethane can be written as follows (the second structure is drawn to show that it is three dimensional):

---

[1] . In the grocery store, "organic" means that the food is grown without artificial pesticides or hormones. The meaning of "organic" in the scientific literature is different from the public literature. In chemistry "organic" is specific to describe carbon-containing molecules. More than one meaning for a word should not confuse us. In life, "love" means "a strong, positive emotion", but in tennis, "love" means "zero".

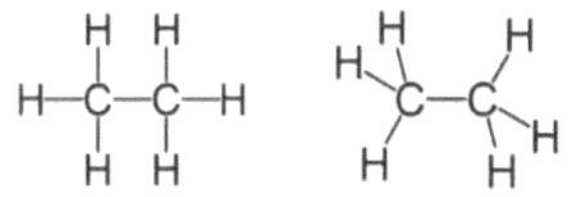

Propane is used as fuel in propane tanks. Propane has three C's and it can be written as:

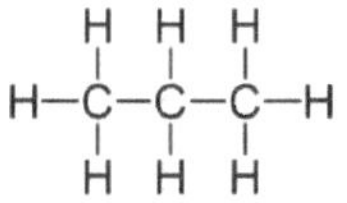

The adjective forms to describe methane, ethane and propane when they are bonded to other molecules are methyl, ethyl and propionyl. So when you see these terms you will know that you are talking about 1, 2 and 3 carbons, respectively.

Three C compounds are the basis of carbohydrates and two C compounds form the building blocks of fats. Our emphasis will be on two and three C compounds, but reference to one C compounds will be found in later chapters.   We already know two one C compounds: CO_2 and urea.

2.3.1 Two carbons

The important molecule that is based upon two C's is acetate. Acetate is:

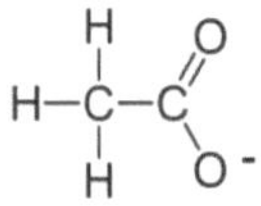

Like ethane, acetate has two carbons, but one carbon has two oxygen atoms on it. This end looks a bit like CO_2 and this end group is called the carboxyl end or carboxylate. Acetate has a negative charge. Like ammonia it can pick up H from water.   Then it becomes acetic acid, and it does not have a charge. Acetic acid is:

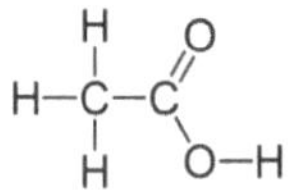

When fat is metabolized in the body it gets broken down to acetate, which then gets converted to CO_2. In this case, acetate is an example of an "intermediary metabolite." It stays within the body and it is not a final metabolite (as is H_2O and CO_2), but acetate is on the pathway of converting fat to CO_2 and H_2O.

Acetic acid and acetate are actual foods. Acetic acid is the major component of vinegar and most salad dressings. As you are reading this, your body is either making acetate or using it. If you have just eaten a big meal, acetate is the building block to make fat, fat being the major storage form of energy. And if you have not eaten for a while, fat is being broken down to acetate. But you may say, "Hey! I don't smell like vinaigrette!" That is because in the body, acetate has a big long tail on it. The tail is called coenzyme A, and it is abbreviated as CoA. Here is acetyl-CoA:

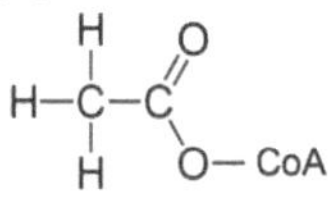

The long CoA keeps the acetate group within the cell. The acetyl part undergoes metabolism to form CO_2. The CoA part gets broken off, and reattached to another acetate molecule. When we talk about acetylCoA, we are really just thinking of the acetate part.

9

2.3.2 Three Carbons

Derivatives of propane are also important intermediary metabolites. A compound similar to acetate is propionate. Propionate and acetate have the same carboxyl end group (COO⁻) but propionate has three C's. Propionate is:

$$
\begin{array}{ccc}
H & H & O \\
| & | & \diagup \\
H-C-C-C & \\
| & | & \diagdown \\
H & H & O^-
\end{array}
$$

In the cell, propionate has CoA attached to it. It is called propionyl CoA. Three carbon molecules based upon propane are intermediates in the metabolism of carbohydrates, i.e., foods like sugar and flour. Pyruvate and lactate are the most common 3 C molecules that are formed in the body from carbohydrates. Pyruvate has one more O and two less H's than propionate:

$$
\begin{array}{ccc}
H & O & O \\
| & \| & \diagup \\
H-C-C-C & \\
| & & \diagdown \\
H & & O^-
\end{array}
$$

Lactate has one more H than pyruvate. This is lactate:

$$
\begin{array}{ccc}
& H & \\
H & O & O \\
| & | & \diagup \\
H-C-C-C & \\
| & | & \diagdown \\
H & H & O^-
\end{array}
$$

The small molecules are summarized in Table 2. Two C and 3 C molecules are the basis of most food.

In Table 2 acetate, pyruvate and lactate are in bold, because they are important in metabolism and will be discussed late. Ethanol is the compound in alcoholic drinks. It is like acetate, but has one fewer oxygen atom. When wine is allowed to sit around, its ethanol gets converted to acetic acid, and the wine tastes terrible. Acetic acid is the main component of vinegar.

10

Table 2. Small molecules: acetate and propionate are building blocks of food

Number C's	Name	Atoms	Structure
1	methane	CH_4	
2	ethane	C_2H_6	
2	ethanol	C_2H_5OH	
2	**acetate**	$C_2H_3O_2$	
3	propane	C_3H_8	
3	**propionate**	$C_3H_5O_2$	
3	**pyruvate**	$C_3H_3O_3$	
3	**lactate**	$C_3H_4O_3$	

2.4 Carbohydrates, fats and proteins are three categories of food

The three types of foods that we digest are carbohydrates, fats and proteins. We also eat fiber. Cellulose is a type of carbohydrate made by plants, but we do not digest it, and cellulose is therefore not food but it is fiber and it passes through our digestive tract and gets excreted in the feces.

Fats, carbohydrates and proteins get much publicity based upon popular diets, where recommendations are given on what you eat and when you eat. An example, the Atkins diet is high in fat and protein. In contrast, a "high carb" diet has little fat but most calories come from carbohydrates.

These diets are often beneficial for some people. For instance, a low protein diet is recommended for people who have types of liver or kidney problems, because urea, the end product of protein, is made in the liver and filtered out of the body in the kidneys. By eating a diet low protein, these organs are spared from having to process a lot of ammonia. On the other hand, a high protein diet may be recommended for a growing child because the child needs extra amino acids from protein to make his or her own proteins. In addition, a high protein diet is often recommended for a burn victim or someone who has been sick for a long time with infection or cancer. These patients need to make proteins in order to restore their tissues.

11

Even a vinegar diet is sometimes touted. Vinegar, which is mostly acetic acid, may clean your coffee pot, but in your body acetic acid supplies calories. If you are not using enough calories, acetic acid in vinegar will be converted to fat.

Sadly, alcohol, i.e. ethanol, is the source of the majority of calories for a few people. Ethanol is a 2 C molecule and, like acetic acids, it is converted into fat by the body. A diet high in ethanol may lack essential nutrients, and excess ethanol has other direct deleterious effects on the body.

2.5 Carbohydrates

Carbohydrates are made up of sugars. We can understand the chemistry of sugar based upon what we already know about molecules. Two versions of the structure of glucose, the most common sugar in the body, are below:

The two ways to write glucose show identical molecules. When sugar is dissolved in water, the cyclic structure occurs. The linear structure on the left is easier to see, so both forms are used in textbooks. What is important is to note that glucose contains six C's. It also has six O's. Five of these O's are in the form of –OH. The –OH group is called hydroxyl.

We have seen –OH before. OH is part of water molecule. So part of glucose is like water – and because of that sugar dissolves well in water. Glucose is the sugar molecule that is in our blood. If your doctor tells you that you have high blood sugar, it means that you have elevated levels of this molecule, glucose, in your blood.

Glucose is a carbohydrate molecule because it is built of C's ("carbo") and OH's (hydrate),[2] The body breaks glucose in half, making two 3 C molecules (pyruvate and/or lactate). Glucose,
therefore, belongs to a class of molecules that are made of three C units.

Glucose is called a mono-saccharide, meaning that it is composed of one sugar molecule. Table sugar and flour are also carbohydrates. The molecules of table sugar are composed of glucose and fructose, two monosaccharides. Because table sugar molecules are composed of two sugar groups, it is called a di-saccharide. Flour is made up of a string of many mono-saccharides. In this case each molecule has so many saccharide groups and so flour is called a polysaccharide. It is also called a complex carbohydrate. Carbohydrates are broken down to mono-saccharides in the intestine, and then they enter the blood circulation. Because it takes more time to break down a

---

[2] Carbo comes from Latin *carbo*, meaning charcoal. Hydrate comes from Greek *hydro*, meaning water. Source: W. S. Haubrich, Medical Meanings. A Glossary of Word Origins, American College of Physicians, 2003.

polysaccharide than a disaccharide, eating a polysaccharide produces a lower spike in blood glucose than when table sugar is eaten.

Carbohydrates are stored in all cells. The form of carbohydrate that is stored in cells is called **glycogen**. Glycogen can be considered the "flour" of humans. Although we all know that we store fat, it may be amazing to learn that our bodies also store "flour," i.e. glycogen. Athletes will sometimes consume carbohydrates before a race to increase the content of glycogen in their muscles. The amount of glycogen stored is not great, but we will see how important it is to allow muscles and brain to function.

In glycogen molecules, sugar molecules are attached to each other to form long strands that have branches in them. In the picture below showing a glycogen molecule, each hexagonal ring represents a sugar molecule, having 6 C's and 6 O's.

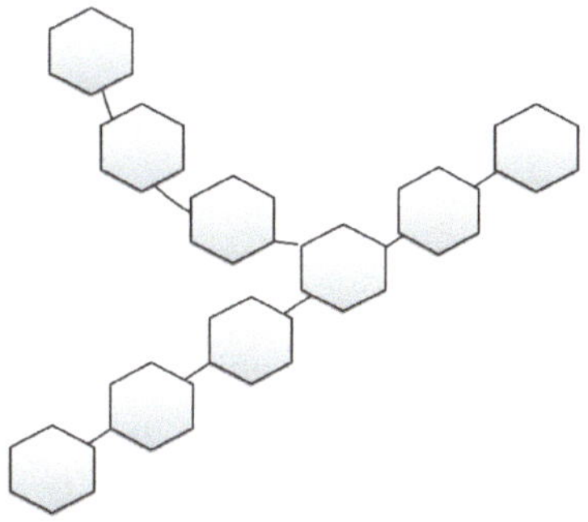

Figure 2.1 Glycogen

Each of the hexagons represents one glucose group. The glucose groups are strung together in a branched arrangement to make glygogen. Thousand of glucose groups are bound together to make glycogen.

In case you are skeptical that flour is made up of sugar, you can do a simple experiment. Chew a soda cracker (made mostly of flour) for a long time. Do you notice that gradually the cracker tastes sweet? That is because the flour is broken down to sugar by the enzyme amylase that is in your saliva. Even as you are chewing you are beginning to digest your food.

Although glucose is the main sugar in blood, there are many types of sugar molecules in the diet. Five C sugars are part of DNA, the genetic material that determines our features and composition of our body.

2.6 Fat

Fat is the major storage form of energy. The word "fat" comes from an old English word *faett*. [3]

The chemical name for fat is triglyceride. To explain this, we distinguish fatty acid and fat. Stearic acid, composed of 18 C's, is the most common fatty acid in our body. Here it is:

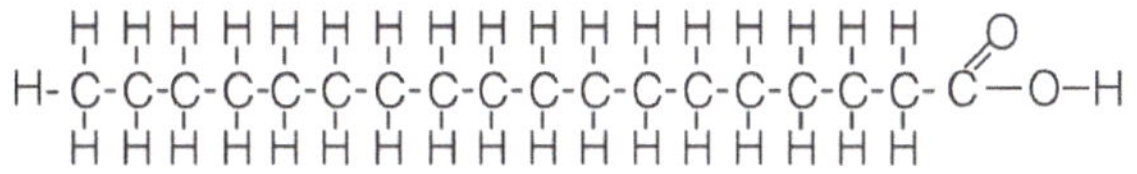

---

[3] Haubrich reports that a related word is "vat", coming from Old English *faet* "vessel."(S. Haubrich, Medical Meaning. A Glossary of Word Origins, American College of Physicians, 2003).

13

Fatty acids are compounds that have a long string of carbons and on one end is a carboxyl group. Chemists often use a shorthand way to write it:

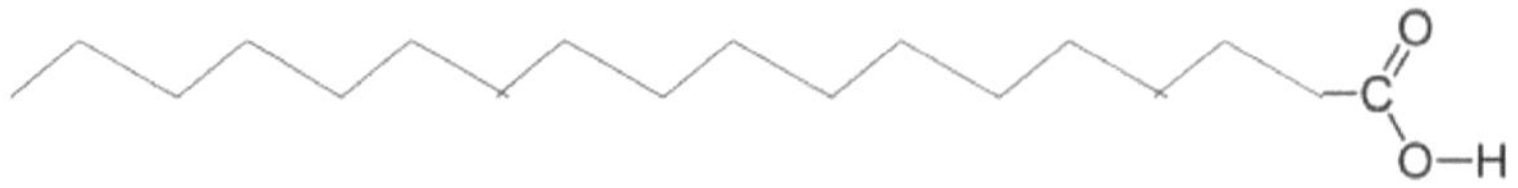

Wherever there is a bend, it is understood that there is a C, and attached to the C are the appropriate number of H's.

Most fatty acids in our body are even numbered. This is because they are made from acetate, which has two carbons. Fatty acids are circulating all the time in our blood.

Fat that we eat, and that is found in our fat tissue is a compound composed of three fatty acids that are hooked together by the molecule glycerol. Glycerol has three carbons and three OH's and is made from glucose. Glycerol is:

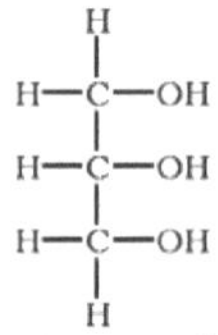

To make fat, a fatty acid molecule bonds to each of the OH's of glycerol. Therefore a fat molecule has three fatty acids.

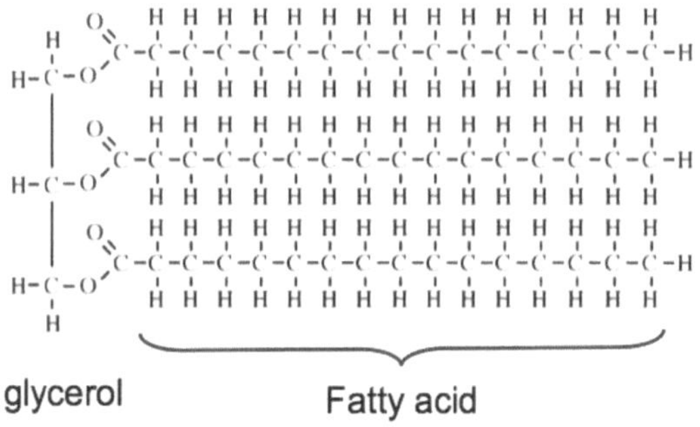

glycerol   Fatty acid

The grocery store sells forms of fat. Olive oil, corn oil, lard and Crisco are all fats. Butter is mostly fat. By definition, fats are composed of fatty acids attached to the three-carbon molecule, glycerol. The different types of fats differ from each other in terms of the composition of the fatty acids. Some of the fatty acids will be long chain and some will be shorter. The 18 C fatty acid is considered long chain, whereas twelve-C fatty acid would be classified as medium chain.

Some fatty acids in fat are "unsaturated." Unsaturated means that not all of the carbons have two H's bonded to them. An example of an unsaturated fatty acid is shown below:

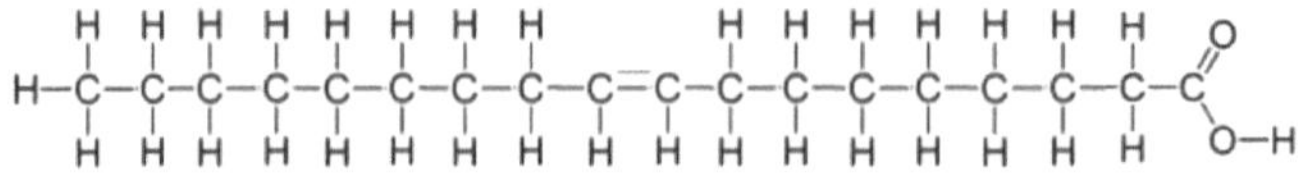

The C=C bond is called an unsaturated bond. The example fatty acid shown above has one unsaturated bond; this fatty acid is a mono-unsaturated fatty acid. More than one bond may be unsaturated. Then the fatty acid is called poly-unsaturated. Unsaturated fats have a lower melting point than saturated fats. At room temperature, olive oil, mostly unsaturated fat, is a liquid, whereas lard, mostly saturated, is a solid. Butter contains more medium chain fatty acids than does lard. The type of fatty acid determines the consistency of fat.

The arrangement of the 2 H's in the double bond is important. As it is shown above, the arrangement is called *cis*. The two H's are on the same side. Our bodies make fatty acids in this arrangement. So do plants and animals. So this is the arrangement found in most of our food. But, in cooking, the consistency of fat is important. To make fat to a harder consistency (desirable for crispness in, say, French fries), H's are chemically added in a process called "hydrogenation". The fatty acid then becomes saturated. This process is never 100%, however. In adding the H to the unsaturated double bond, the bond is ruptured. In a small percentage of the fatty acids the H's then revert to being unsaturated and about 50% of these become trans. This is a trans fatty acid:

Since trans fatty acids are not normally found in large amounts in natural foods, there is a concern that they might not be healthy.

2.7 Proteins

Most reactions in the body require the action of proteins, which act as catalysts to make reactions go faster. Such proteins are called **enzymes**.

Proteins that we eat as food are broken down into individual amino acids and then reused by the body to make proteins that exist in every cell and its surrounding fluids. Amino acids are also used to provide energy for the cell by being broken down to CO_2 and H_2O. Excess amino acids are converted into fat. Unlike fat, which cannot be made into glucose, amino acids can be converted into glucose. This is an important function, since brain needs glucose for fuel.

Proteins are constantly being made and broken down. The excess of N from the amino acids is excreted as urea in the urine.

2.7.1 Proteins are made of amino acids

The word protein comes from the Greek word *proteios* meaning origin or chief.[4] This word reflects the importance of proteins to life.

Proteins are made up of amino acids. "Amino" sounds a bit like "ammonia," which is no coincidence because amino acids contain N. DNA, the genetic material determines the sequence of 20 types of amino acid in our proteins. The simplest amino acid is glycine:

Glycine illustrates how putting together small molecules makes a new molecule. Glycine has two carbon atoms, as does ethane. It has a C with two O's, like carbon dioxide. The –

---

4 The word "protein" was introduced by the Dutch chemist, Gerard Johann Mulder in 1838 (S. Haubrich, Medical meanings. A Glossary of Word Origins, American College of Physicians, 2003).

COOH group is the carboxyl group or carboxylate. In this way, glycine is the same as acetate. But glycine also has –NH$_2$, like ammonia,

Alanine is the most common amino acid in the body. It has 3 C's and its structure is:

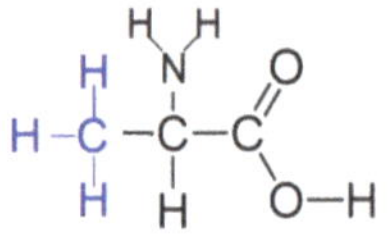

It is a derivative of propane. Note that the parts of glycine and alanine are identical. But, alanine has a methyl group in the place where there is an H in glycine. For the 20 kinds of amino acids in our body, the part of the figure containing the two C to the right is identical for all, whereas the part is different.

Other three C amino acids are serine:

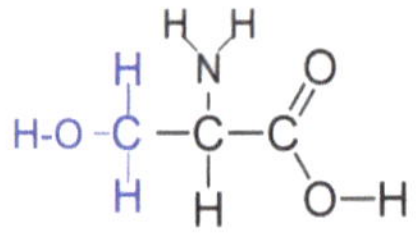

and cysteine:

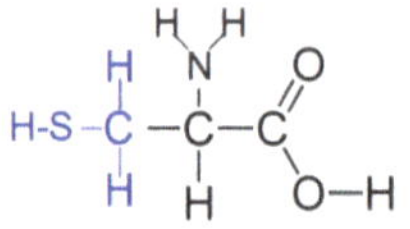

Serine has an OH group on it. This makes it more like water, and it is more soluble in water than is alanine. Cysteine has a new element in it, sulfur, S. The SH group has some special chemistry associated with it; we will learn about this in Chapter 8.

2.7.2 How amino acids join together to make a protein

Amino acids are joined together to make proteins. The carboxyl group of one amino acid combines with the amino group of another amino acid to form a bond.

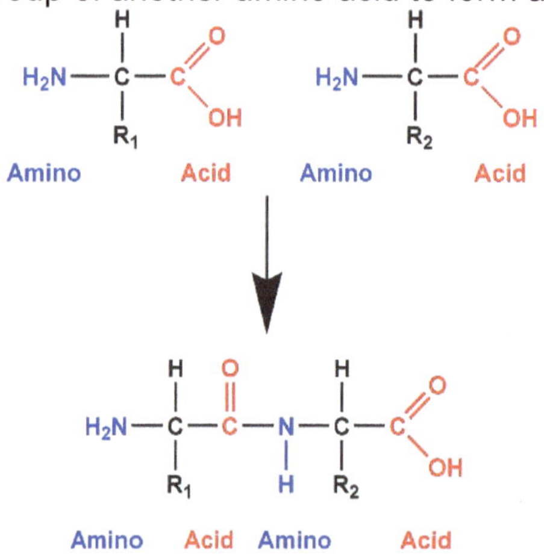

Proteins can be made up of chains of hundreds and even thousands of amino acids. The types of amino acids in the protein and the order in which the amino acids are in the chain determine the characteristics of protein. Hemoglobin, which carries O$_2$ in blood, is a protein. Hair on your head is made from protein. You recognize how different hemoglobin and hair are in function.

2.7.3 Proteins have defined 3-dimensional structures

Muscle is mainly made of proteins that allow us to move. Every tissue in the body contains proteins. The amino acid sequence of a protein determines its function and in humans there are perhaps about 20,000 or more different sequences, and hence different proteins.

Although amino acids combine in a linear fashion – one amino attaches to another and so on, and there are usually no branches like in glycogen, the linear "rope" of amino acids fold to form definite three dimensional structures. The structures of such molecules are complicated, but they have simplifying structural features. There are several folding patterns found in most proteins. One of the most common is the α-helix. An α-helix is illustrated in Figure 2.2 center, where about 14 amino acids coil up to form a helix.

Figure 2.2

Center: 14 to 15 amino acids coil to form a helix. The outline of the helix is shown in red. The small balls represent the atoms of the amino acids.

Right: Example of a protein molecule. This molecule is albumin and it is found in blood plasma.

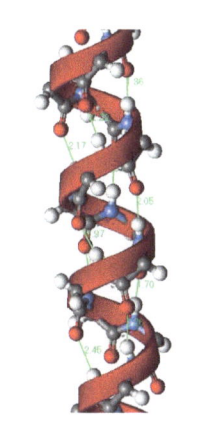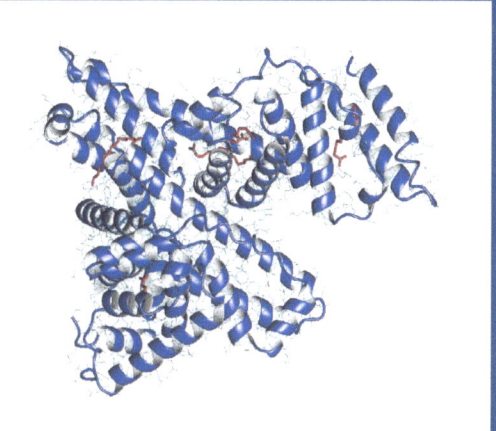

The right panel of Figure 2.2 shows the protein molecule, albumin. Albumin is found in blood plasma. It has nearly 600 amino acids, and you see that it is a very "curly" molecule, having about 20 α-helix portions.

When the amino acids are folded properly, the protein is said to be "native." Native proteins are functional. The function of the albumin molecule is to bind and transport fatty acids in blood plasma.

When protein loses shape and the amino acids are no longer folded in the right way to be functional, the protein is "denatured." Heating, as in cooking, denatures proteins. A cooked egg consists of denatured proteins, and has a different appearance from a raw egg. Denatured proteins retain the same the same amino acids as native proteins and they have the same nutritional value.

Proteins are found in plants and animals. When we eat protein, the protein is broken down to amino acids in the digestive system. Therefore, animal and plant proteins are equally healthy to eat, provided that the proteins contain the amino acids that we require.

2.8 Summary of molecules of metabolism

The beginning of metabolism is food and O_2 and the final end molecules are CO_2, H_2O and urea. Our patient, GB, breathes in air that supplies O_2 to GB.

Figure 2.3. What goes in

Food contains C, H, O and N. Oxygen, O_2, enters the body by breathing.

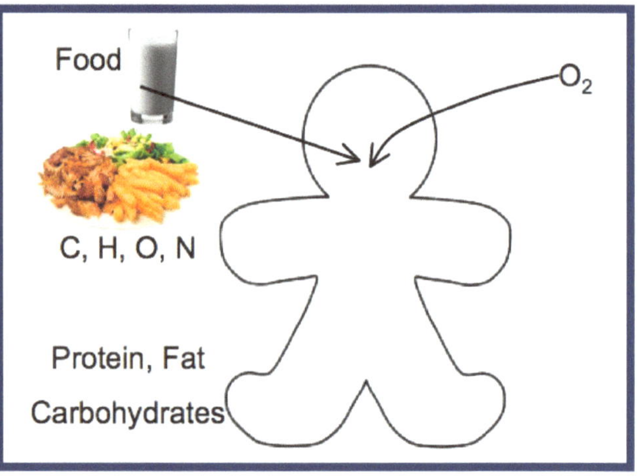

Food

O_2

C, H, O, N

Protein, Fat

Carbohydrates

Food and air are required for energy. In Figure 2.4 GB is running, which consumes more food (calories) and oxygen than when GB is sitting on the couch. During running GB breathes faster to get more O_2. The food and oxygen are transformed to the final products of metabolism. GB breathes CO_2 out from the lungs. H_2O, water, is part of the total water in the body. Water is excreted in urine, lost in sweat and through the lungs. The nitrogen of protein is excreted as urea. Figure 2.4 shows the products of metabolism.

Figure 2.4. What goes out.

Final products of metabolism are small molecules. We breathe out CO_2 in the lungs. H_2O goes into the pool of water in our body and it is excreted in urine, in sweating and through breathing. The element N comes from eating protein. Extra N is excreted in the urine as urea.

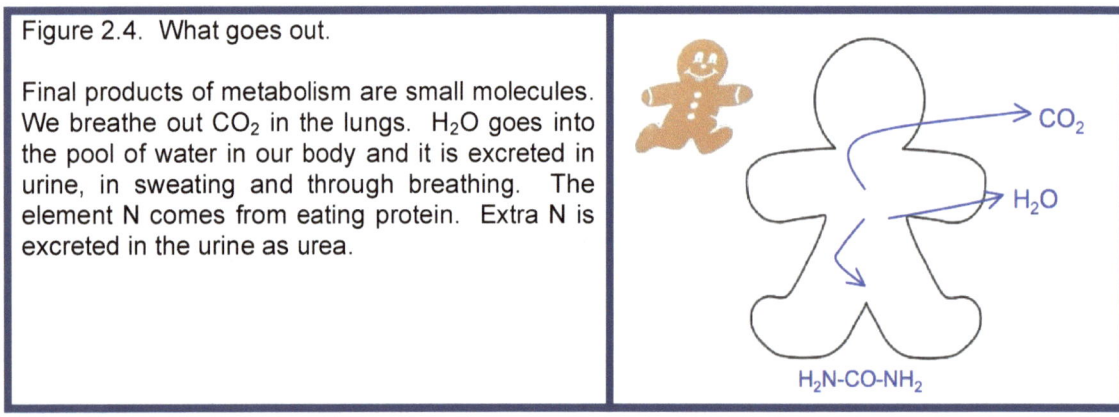

CO_2

H_2O

$H_2N-CO-NH_2$

Metabolism goes on at all times during life. But GB does not eat all of the time. So GB stores food. Food is stored in three ways in the body, shown in Figure 2.5. The most important storage form, where most of the excess carbons are stored, is fat. GB eats fat, carbohydrate or protein, and if GB eats too much of any of these, the body converts the excess C's into fat, and GB becomes obese. A small, but important part of storage is glycogen. Glycogen is like flour and it is found in every tissue of the body, but the most glycogen is found in liver and muscle. In the picture GB is shown with a muscular arm. The purpose of muscles is to do work. But, muscles are also metabolized under some conditions. During fasting or starvation, proteins in our muscles are broken down to form amino acids, which then are used for energy and are metabolized to CO_2, H_2O and urea. The amino acids from protein are made into sugar that the brain needs for energy.

18

| Figure 2.5. Storage forms of food.

1. **Fat** is the largest storage form.
2. **Glycogen** is carbohydrate. Every cell stores glycogen, but the organs with the largest storage of glycogen are liver and muscles.
3. **Proteins** are also used for energy. Proteins are found throughout the body. The largest amount of protein is found in muscles. | 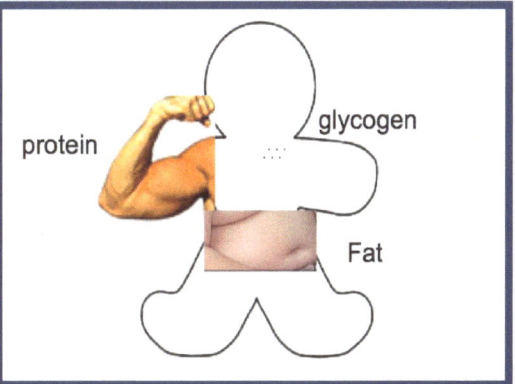 |

When food is not available (during famine) or absorption of food becomes severely limited (during disease), eventually many proteins from the heart and diaphragm are metabolized, and GB will no longer be able to breathe or the heart will not pump. GB and we must eat in order to live.

3. Machinery of a factory: The cell

3.1 ATP provides energy

In the last chapter we introduced the chemical units of molecules that are the basis of our food. Molecules of food are used to make energy. The molecule that provides energy is ATP. The chemical structure of ATP is given later in this chapter. Tissues of the body are composed of cells and ATP is found within every cell.

Let us make a mechanical analogy. Consider a factory making a car. Raw material goes into the factory, and a car comes out. Work is done on the raw material, most of the work being done using electricity. Intelligence is needed to properly assemble the parts, and humans supply this intelligence. To make the car, more than one factory is used. Parts may be made in Kentucky, Japan, Germany, China or other places. Each of these factories requires electricity to power them. And the production in one factory must be correlated with the production in other factories. If hubcaps made at one-factory lags in production, the production of the whole car will be slowed down.

ATP is like the electricity that runs each factory. Electricity must be constantly supplied at a certain level in each factory. When the electricity stops, the production in that factory stops. The overall assembly of cars in another factory will be affected. Like electricity, the amount of ATP in a cell is low, but it must be constantly supplied. If ATP levels drop, the tissue is no longer able to function and it will die.

Unlike a factory, where electricity can be supplied from the outside, every one of the trillion or so cells in the body must make its own ATP. For all the cells to work harmoniously so the whole body functions properly, there must be a way for the production of energy to be regulated in every cell.

Enzymes are proteins that make reactions go faster. Enzymes control the rate that fuel is being used for energy within each cell. Some enzymes are inhibited when metabolites get high. The product of one enzyme is transformed by another enzyme and so on, so that fuel is broken down. In this way enzymes work together to form a pathway, changing one metabolite into another.

But, the rate that food is used, also needs to be controlled by means outside of the cell.

There are several ways that cells communicate with each other. One way is by **hormones**. Hormones are chemicals that are produced in one part of the body that regulate the cells in other tissues. Hormones control the reactions of most enzymatic pathways. Hormones are the means that the actions of cells in one tissue are correlated with the function of another tissue.

Some pathways are regulated by **innervation**. The brain sends an electrical signal via the nerves to trigger the action of a certain pathway.

3.2 Cells

All of our tissues are composed of cells, and as we mentioned we have about a trillion cells. (A large person has more cells than a small person). A simplified cell is shown in Figure 3.1:

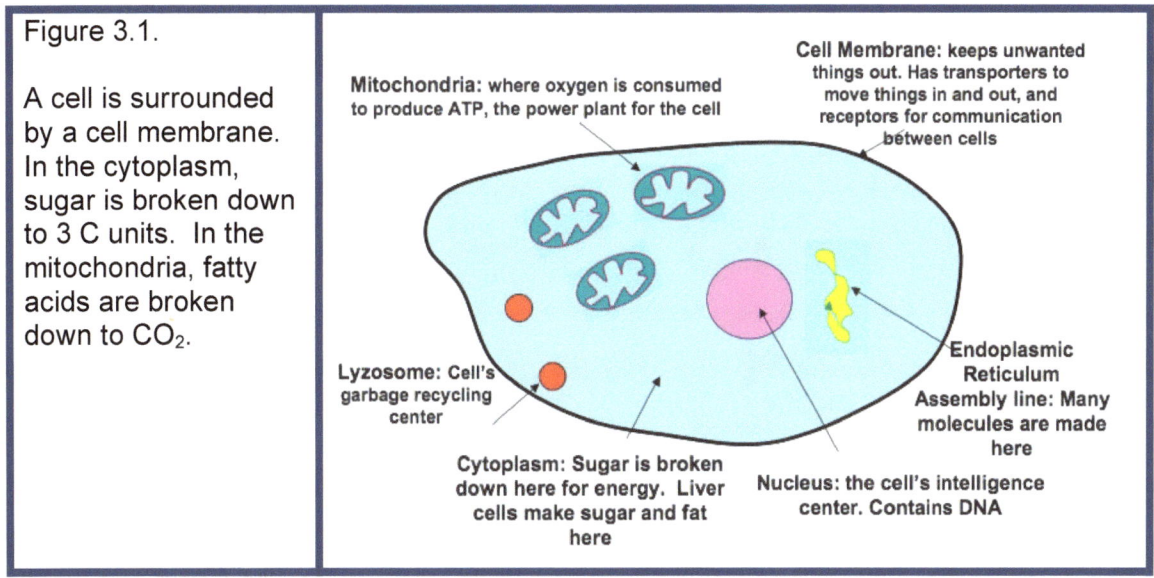

Figure 3.1.

A cell is surrounded by a cell membrane. In the cytoplasm, sugar is broken down to 3 C units. In the mitochondria, fatty acids are broken down to CO_2.

Mitochondria: where oxygen is consumed to produce ATP, the power plant for the cell

Cell Membrane: keeps unwanted things out. Has transporters to move things in and out, and receptors for communication between cells

Lyzosome: Cell's garbage recycling center

Cytoplasm: Sugar is broken down here for energy. Liver cells make sugar and fat here

Nucleus: the cell's intelligence center. Contains DNA

Endoplasmic Reticulum Assembly line: Many molecules are made here

To supply a factory, raw materials must go in, and the product of the factory must come out. The same is true of the cell. Surrounding the cell is the cell membrane; it is like the wall around factory with gates to control access to the factory. Nutrients go into the cell across this membrane and by-products of metabolism go out in a controlled manner. Only some things have a "tracking number" enabling it to go in or out of the cell. The "gates" for cell membranes are specialized transporter molecules. The cell must communicate with other cells. Receptor molecules in the cell membrane recognize hormones that signal from the outside for changes to occur in the inside.

Within the cell certain things occur only at defined locations. DNA resides in the **nucleus**. Information in DNA determines the sequence of all of the proteins that are made in our body. It is what makes each of us unique.

The **endoplasmic reticulum** is an organelle composed of membranes within the cell. Proteins and other molecules are made and modified on these membranes. You can think of the endoplasmic reticulum as making the enzymes, which are the "machinery" for metabolism.

Within another membrane structure, the **lyzosome**, many molecules are degraded. The lyzosome is analogous to the garbage-recycling center.

In the next chapters, metabolism that occurs in the **cytoplasm** and **mitochondria** will be described. In the cytoplasm sugars are metabolized to three carbon units. In the mitochondria three carbon molecules (mostly from sugar) and two carbon molecules (mostly from fat) are transformed to CO_2 and water by reacting with O_2. In the reactions occurring in the cytoplasm and mitochondria all of the cell's ATP is produced. Most of the ATP is made by mitochondria -- the power generators of the cell.

3.3. Membranes separate compartments of cells

Cells are beautiful things. They do many things – all at once. For instance they may be consuming ATP to make proteins at the same time they are using fat to make ATP. In order to do many things at once reactions must be separated from each other. Membranes accomplish this separation. Substances inside of the must not leak out. Again membranes keep what should be inside from leaking out. What are biological membranes?

One of the major components of membranes is lecithin. Lecithin is very similar to fat. You remember that fat is composed of three fatty acids bound to the three OH's of glycerol. Lecithin has two fatty acids bound to glycerol. On the third OH of glycerol is a substance called choline.

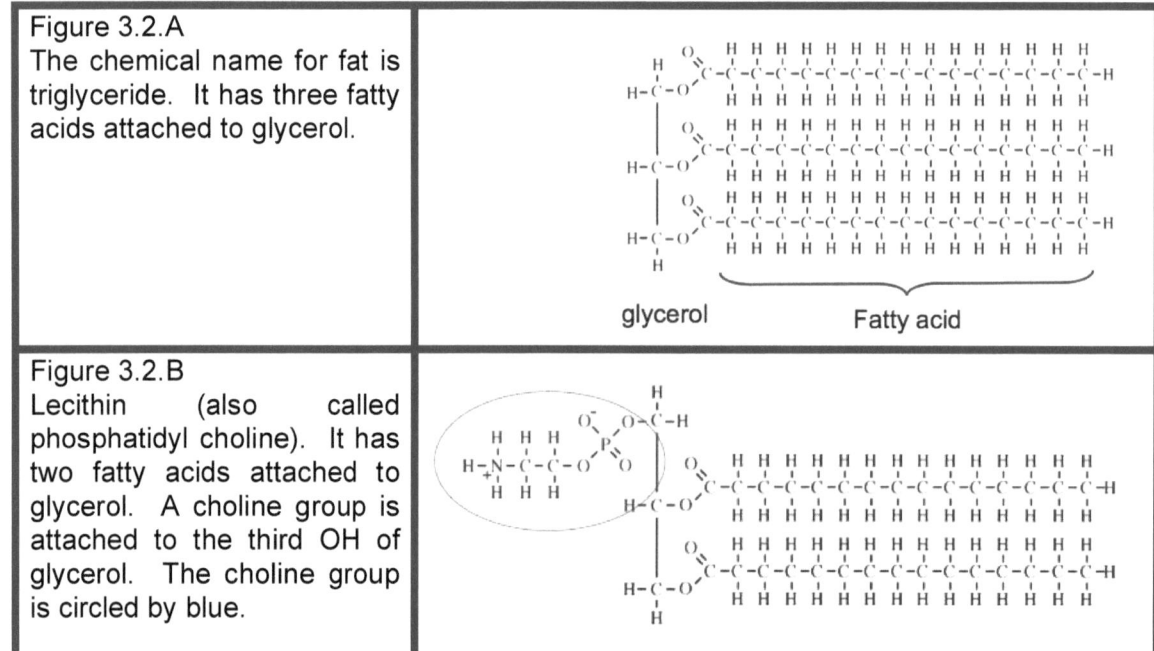

| Figure 3.2.A
The chemical name for fat is triglyceride. It has three fatty acids attached to glycerol. | |
| Figure 3.2.B
Lecithin (also called phosphatidyl choline). It has two fatty acids attached to glycerol. A choline group is attached to the third OH of glycerol. The choline group is circled by blue. | |

Choline has a positive charge on the N, and a negative charge on the phosphate. This group is hydrophilic, meaning that it likes water. The fatty acid part is hydrophobic, meaning it does not like water.

Lecithin molecules associate with each other so that the fatty acids are oriented away from the water, and the choline is in the water. By so doing, the lecithin makes a membrane. There are two sides: an inside and an outside, both exposed to water. The choline group is called the head group, and the fatty acids are called the tails. This is shown in Figure 3.3

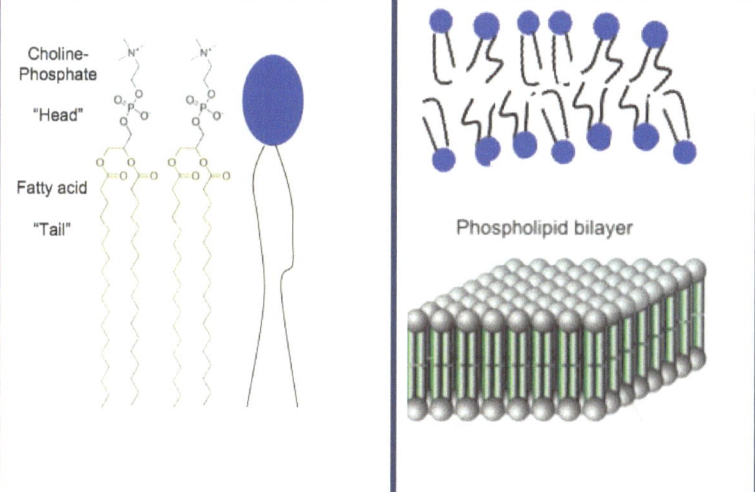

Figure 3.3

Middle panel: Phosphatidyl choline molecules interact with each other so that hydrophobic part – the fatty acids – interact with each other. The choline part is hydrophilic (water loving) and this part associates with water.

Right panel: The phospholipids molecules form two layers, with water being on either side.

Biological membranes are composed of lecithin plus many other compounds similar to lecithin. Instead of the "choline" part, there may be a compound resembling an amino acid or sugar. When the head group is sugar, the compound is called a glycolipid. Glycolipids are found in high amounts in nerve cells. There are a large number of different types of lipids in membranes. Membranes have different lipids within them. Unsaturated lipids are fluid, and they keep the center, hydrophobic part, flexible. We cannot make lipids that have many unsaturated double bonds, and we must get them from our diet.

Embedded into the bilayer of lipids are proteins. The blobs in Figure 3.4 represent proteins. Some proteins go across the membranes. Ion pumps and receptor molecules have one part of them on the outside.. Other proteins are attached to one side of the membrane or the other.

Figure 3.4 A membrane

The lecithin and other phosphatidyl compounds form two layers, with water on both sides of the membrane. Some protein molecules (shown as aqua) go across the membrane; others are attached to either the inside or outside (shown as pink).

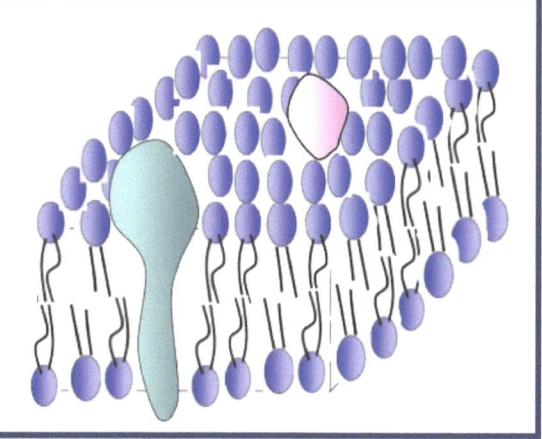

Many enzymes are located on or in membranes, and therefore many reactions in cells occur at membrane surfaces.

3.4 ATP is the energy unit of the cell

We introduced a new term – ATP. ATP is a molecule that gives the energy used to power everything the cell does. But then we have the question: what is the energy? This may seem like a deep philosophical question – and indeed it is! (Who am I? What is matter? What is energy?) However, the answer is simple for living systems. Most energy that is used for all cells comes from the molecule ATP. The full name of ATP is adenosine triphosphate.

ATP is composed of N, H, C's. (Remember that wherever there is a bend in the structure, there is a C with its attached H's.) It also contains a new element phosphorous, P. In fact, it has three P's, and hence it is called triphosphate. This is ATP:

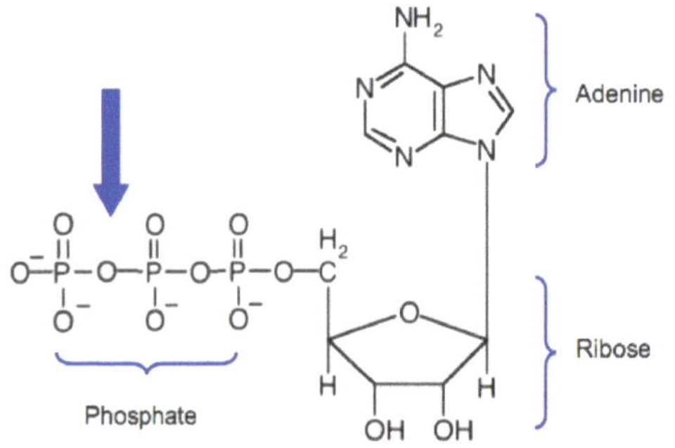

ATP is made of three parts: adenine, ribose (a sugar) and phosphate groups. The thing that you should know is that the business end of ATP deals with the element phosphorous, denoted as P. P is bonded to oxygen, O, as shown in the figure, and oxygen and phosphorous together is called phosphate. The bond indicated by the blue arrow is especially unstable. This bond produces energy when it is broken. When the cell needs energy, the phosphate (P and O) comes off, and energy is produced. The amount of energy is described in calories. One mole of phosphate coming off of ATP gives about 10 calories of energy. (A mole tells the number of molecules. One mole is 602,000,000,000,000,000,000,000 molecules.[1] Since it takes too much time to write this big number, the term mole is used.)

 ATP that loses one phosphate becomes ADP (adenosine diphosphate). ADP is shown below. It is identical to ATP but has two phosphate groups rather than three.

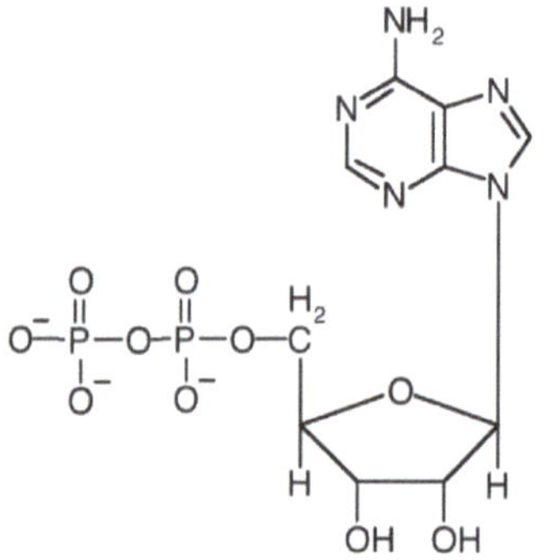

During metabolism of food, ATP is formed from ADP. When the cell needs energy ATP breaks down to ADP. An adult person has about 0.1 mole of ATP in the body. But an adult uses about 200 moles of ATP every day. ADP must be constantly be made back into ATP. This is what food does. It makes ATP from ADP, constantly supplying the body with energy.

---

[1] In scientific notation this number is 6.02×10^{23}.

3.5 Every cell must make its own ATP

A factory in France does not share its electricity with a factory in Dubai. Each factory must have its own energy source. Likewise, cells do not share ATP molecules. ATP is *inside* cells, not in blood or other fluids surrounding cells. The membrane surrounding the cell does not allow ATP to leak out into blood.

It then follows: *each and every cell uses energy from its own ATP and uses its own metabolism to remake ATP from ADP.*

There are a few reactions in the cell that derive their energy from compounds other than ATP, but for species on earth the overwhelming source of energy is ATP.   ATP is so universally found in life species, that the presence of ATP was used as a biomarker to search for life on Mars.   The thinking is that if life forms on Mars and on Earth have common origins, then Martian life will also use ATP for energy.

3.6 Why does every cell need ATP (energy)?

Cells use ATP to "buy" various actions that occur in the cell. What are the uses of ATP in the cell?

3.6.1 Energy is required to keep the ions (aka "electrolytes") in the proper concentration

Table salt is sodium chloride (NaCl) and when it dissolves into water it becomes the ions Na^+ (sodium) and Cl^- (chloride), where Na^+ and the Cl^- are separate from each other. Blood plasma has Na^+ and Cl^- in it; in fact blood plasma is about as salty as ocean water. Whereas blood plasma and the fluids around cells are high in Na^+, inside of the cell there is another ion, potassium (K^+).   Nerve cells especially need the proper salt concentration. Your brain will not function if too much Na comes into the cells and too much K^+ comes out. The heart will not beat if K^+ levels in the blood get too high.

At all times some of the K^+ leaks out of the cell and Na^+ leaks in through the cell membrane. To keep Na^+ out and K^+ in requires energy. This is illustrated in Figure 3.5.

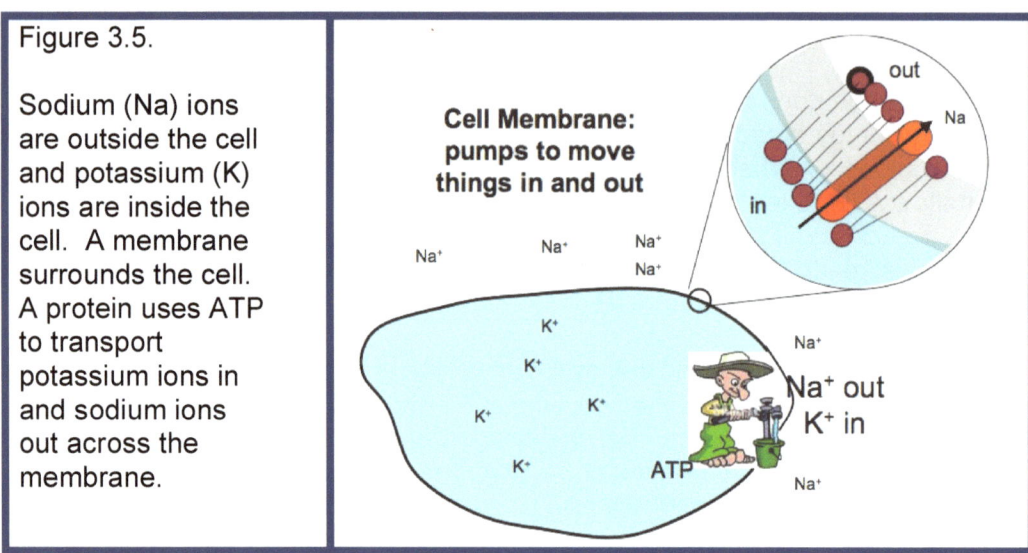

Figure 3.5.

Sodium (Na) ions are outside the cell and potassium (K) ions are inside the cell. A membrane surrounds the cell. A protein uses ATP to transport potassium ions in and sodium ions out across the membrane.

Cell Membrane: pumps to move things in and out

Na$^+$ out
K$^+$ in

Figure 3.5 shows a little guy pumping Na$^+$ out and K$^+$ in. Of course, there is no "little guy" in your cell membranes. The pumps really are proteins in the cell membrane. The inset shows a magnification of the cell membrane. Na and K ions cannot go through the fatty acid part of lecithin very well. The red cylinder, representing a pump or transporter molecule, is a protein. Pumps take Na that is inside the cell and moves it to the outside to the blood plasma. Other pumps take K that is outside and move it inside. Just like the little man needs to exert energy to work his pump, the pumps that transport ions need to accomplish their tasks. That energy is comes from ATP; it releases energy when the phosphate detaches, the ion is transported and ATP becomes ADP.

Because the K that is inside of the cell gradually leaks out and Na gradually leaks in, the pumps have to be working all the time. So metabolism occurs all the time to transform ADP back into ATP. A large percentage of basal metabolism – the amount of food used when you are not exercising – is used to maintain ion levels in cells

Blood plasma is high in calcium (Ca^{++}) and phosphate. Ca^{++} and phosphate are found in bone, but all cells require them. Ca and P have separate pumps, i.e. proteins in the membrane that are transporters. Basically, all substances that the cell needs have transporters or pumps to bring the substance into the cell, and transporters also take substances that are products of metabolism from inside the cell and deposit these chemicals into the blood.

3.6.2 ATP is needed for cell division. DNA is in the nucleus. During growth, each of our chromosomes containing DNA gets replicated and the cell divides to make a new cell. Many cells and proteins are as old as we are. The proteins that are in the center of your eye lens are as old as you are. Some cells, such as nerves and muscles, do not often form new cells in an adult. Although the proteins within these cells are constantly being degraded and reformed, the cell itself does not often multiply to make new cells to replace old cells. Other cells are being formed and removed from our body constantly. An example is red blood cells. Red blood cells last around 120 days in the blood; then they are removed from the blood by the spleen. The body is constantly making new red blood cells. Cells in the intestinal wall are also constantly regenerating, and skin cells are constantly being shed, and remade. The constant formation of new cells requires cell division and, hence, energy.

There are conditions when the body needs to make many new cells. During a child's growth spurt, the parents are aware that suddenly the child is eating them out of house and home. Milk, bread, everything suddenly disappear from the refrigerator. The calorie intake is very large. Burn victims also need to synthesize new tissue. A high protein, high calorie diet is often recommended for these patients. When you get a little paper cut on your finger, cells die and the body repairs the cut by making more cells. Energy is needed! After major surgery or severe infection, more mending is needed. More cells are destroyed and more need to be remade. Making new cells requires much energy.

3.6.3 ATP is needed to synthesize molecules. Not only are whole cells dying and being regenerated, but also protein, fat and glycogen molecules within cells are being degraded and remade. The old adage is, "You are what you eat" is not true! In fact, that carrot that you are eating contains its own DNA, proteins and membranes. Carrot DNA and protein molecules do not become your DNA and proteins. Your cells make complicated molecules and structures like DNA and proteins, fat and glucose from simple molecules. The synthesis of complicated molecules takes energy.

3.6.4 ATP is needed for motion; muscles use ATP during exercise. Running, jumping, walking and all exercise activities require many calories, supplied by many ATP molecules. A training athlete may use 4000 Kcal (kilocalories) and about 3000 of these calories are used for motion. Most diet regimens suggest exercise along with reduced calories to lose weight.

3.7 Cells and organs are specialized

The metabolism of cells and tissues is specialized and one tissue may need more ATP than another tissue at a given time. The brain always needs ATP, since it constantly needs to maintain ions such as Na and K at the right levels. The brain is somewhat unique as a tissue because it does not use fat as a fuel. It uses carbohydrates, although there is an exception – during long term starvation a product of fat is used, which we will discuss later.

In chapter 1, we considered what happens in a brain after eating sugar and during fasting. In contrast to the brain, muscles do not need much ATP when they are resting. But they suddenly need energy during exercise. The diagram explains what occurs in muscle.

Figure 3.6 After GB eats carbohydrates, sugar circulates in the blood. Muscles take up some of the sugar and transform the sugar into glycogen. This glycogen is stored in muscle.

During strenuous exercise muscle glycogen is broken down to 6 C sugar (glucose-phosphate) and then to 3 C. In this process ATP is formed to provide energy for the muscle. The final 3 C compound formed in muscle is lactate.

During less strenuous exercise, muscle uses fat and O_2 to form ATP.

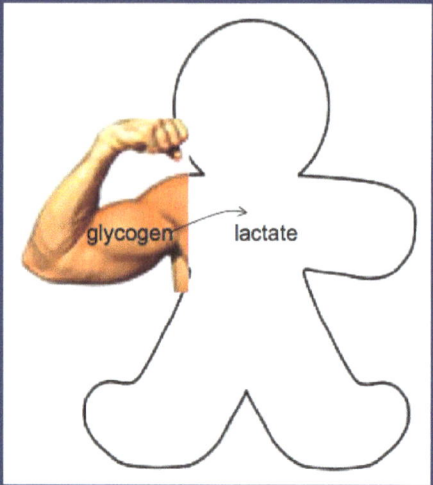

glycogen   lactate

Exercise illustrates how various organs interact. When glucose is high in blood, muscle uses glucose from blood for energy. Muscle also stores glycogen and it breaks down to form glucose that gets broken down to 3 C compounds, namely pyruvate and lactate. Metabolism of glucose and glycogen to form pyruvate and lactate produces ATP, and does not require O_2.

Fat is also used by muscle to form ATP, but the use of fat requires O_2. So glycogen and glucose are used when exercise is so rigorous that O_2 supplied to the muscle does not keep up with the demand for ATP.

The muscle will use up the produced lactate during anerobic (fast) exercise, if after a vigorous work-out, exercise is continued slowly so that O_2 is delivered to the muscle and the muscle continues to work. This is the rationale for the "cool down" phase on exercise machines. If you suddenly stop exercising, the lactate stays in the muscle, but it gradually leaks out, and the liver ultimately metabolizes it to CO_2. In the meantime, however, your muscles may be feeling a bit sore.

3.8 Metabolism is regulated: how cells and organs communicate with each other

You may be getting a feeling of the marvelous engine that is the human body. Instead of one motor, every cell makes its own ATP. But, if you are hungry, it does not mean that all your tissues and cells need nourishment. The metabolism of every single cell in every tissue is regulated so that the right thing is happening at the right time.

The human body is complicated and there are many levels of regulation of metabolism.

3.8.1 One level of regulation occurs within cells. Enzymes are specialized protein molecules found in all cells. (All enzymes are proteins, but not all proteins are enzymes). Enzymes catalyze all reactions in the body and we have thousands of enzymes. Enzymes determine the speed that a reaction will go. For life to be maintained there must always a flux of metabolites. Some are going into the cell, ATP is being generated and the waste products are going out.

How enzymes work is that they bind a metabolite, and then the reaction occurs at a cleft on the enzyme surface.   Since the regulation of glucose levels is such an important part of metabolism we use glucokinase as an illustration for an enzyme.   Glucokinase catalyzes (i.e. makes go faster) the reaction in which a phosphate from ATP gets attached to glucose:

ATP + glucose → glucose-6-phosphate + ADP

Figure 3.7. A picture of a molecule of the enzyme, glucokinase. In this picture, the blue parts are the string of amino acids that make up the protein part of glucokinase. Green is ATP and yellow is glucose. Glucose and ATP bind to the protein part of glucokinase.	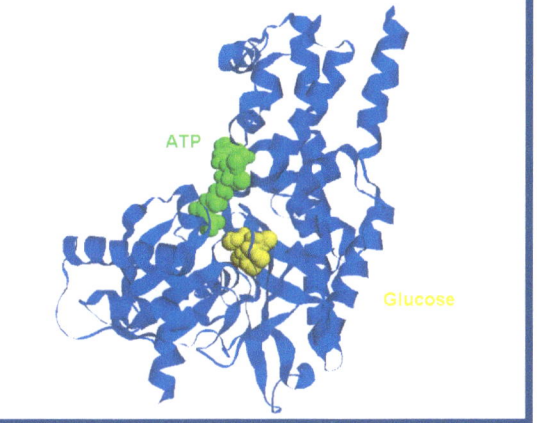

After glucose enters the cell, glucokinase is the first enzyme that reacts with the metabolite glucose. Glucose binds to glucokinase and then ATP binds. The adenine and ribose part of the molecule (see the structure given above) serve to anchor ATP to the enzyme, glucokinase.   Within milliseconds after glucose and ATP binds, a phosphate gets transferred to glucose. ATP becomes ADP. Glucose becomes glucose-6-phosphate. Then both ADP and glucose-6-phosphate are released from the enzyme.

Enzymes make reactions go much faster than the reaction would go without the enzyme. Without the enzyme the reaction may take several years, with it, the reaction is completed in less than a second.   Glucose-6-phosphate can not cross the cell membrane; it is trapped in the cell, and other enzymes ultimately act to break it down to give energy to the cell.

If glucose-6-6phosphate concentrations get high, it will stay bound to the enzyme and the enzyme will no longer be able to bind glucose, and the enzyme will no longer be able to put phosphate on. When the enzyme is no longer able to work, we say that the enzyme is inhibited. Glucose-6--phosphate is an inhibitor of the enzyme glucokinase. This prevents too much glucose from entering the cell.

Some enzymes bind other substances too.   These substances can activate enzymes or inhibit. Products of the reactions often inhibit. Then when too much product builds up, the enzyme will not work as well; this prevents more product being formed.   This kind of inhibition is called feed-back inhibition.

3.8.2 Hormones regulate metabolism. Superimposed upon the regulation of metabolism at the cellular level by enzymes, there are there is a more general regulation by hormones. Hormones are chemical compounds that are made in one organ, but affect the metabolism within cells of other organs.

Many hormones do not go into the cell, but they regulate what is going on inside by binding to the outside of the cell membrane. Insulin is one such hormone.

When glucose in the blood is high, the pancreas secretes insulin into the blood. Therefore, in normal conditions when blood glucose is high, the blood insulin level is also high. Insulin binds to a receptor in the cell membrane. Receptor is like a traffic light; it tells some reactions in the cell to "go" and others to slow down or stop. This shown in the scheme showed on Figure 3.8. The receptors acts indirectly by activating an enzyme that takes ATP to put a phosphate on a specific amino acid of important enzymes. This enzyme then changes other enzymes. One such protein that is changed is the transporter of the sugar glucose. In this case, the binding of insulin to the insulin receptor triggers the removal of glucose from blood, and transport into the cell.

Figure 3.8

All cell membranes have insulin receptors. Insulin receptors act as traffic lights, telling some reactions to go faster, and other reactions to go slower. Insulin receptors are proteins that bind insulin. When insulin is bound to the outside of the cell, the part of the receptor that is inside triggers a reaction that takes a phosphate from ATP and attaches to specific proteins. One protein that is ultimately affected is the glucose transporter. When insulin binds to the receptor, the transporter is active, and it transports glucose from blood into the cell.

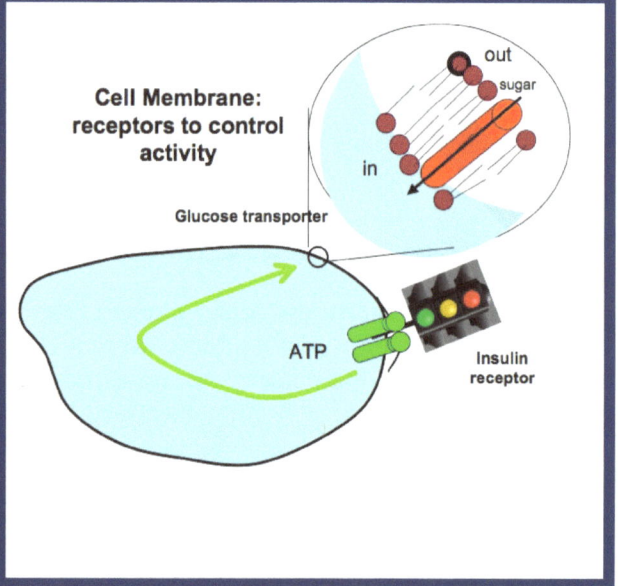

Insulin is a major hormone that regulates overall metabolism. It serves to remove glucose, fat and amino acids from the blood.   Insulin is a protein; it is made of amino acids.   It is one of several hormones made in the pancreas. All cells have insulin receptors. In Figure 3.10, arrows show how insulin is affecting various organs.

| Figure 3.9.

 The effects of insulin are wide-ranging. It stimulates muscle and other tissues to take in glucose from the blood plasma. Insulin stimulates protein synthesis of muscle. It stimulates glycogen and fat synthesis in the liver. Fat transport from the liver to adipose (fat) tissue is stimulated by insulin. | 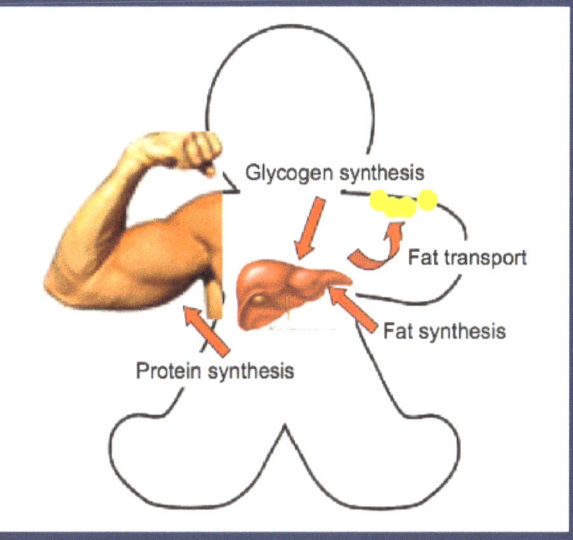 |

High insulin stimulates glycogen synthesis and fat synthesis in the liver, and the transport of fat to adipose (fat) tissue. It also stimulates protein synthesis in muscle and other tissues. All cells in the body have receptors for insulin. The over-arching effect of insulin is to stimulate enzymes that act to store fuel, and inhibit enzymes that release fuel from glycogen and fat stores.

3.8.3 Nervous system also regulates metabolism

Many additional hormones are involved in the regulation of metabolism. Cortisol, adrenaline (also called epinephrine) and glucogon are hormones that serve to mobilize stored fats, carbohydrates and proteins and thereby restore glucose levels. The production of adrenaline is controlled by the nervous system.

Our patient GB is walking on a path through the woods. Suddenly a great big ugly brown bear jumps out in front of GB. What happens to GB? His brain signals the adrenal gland to make adrenaline. The adrenal gland is found on top of the kidneys. Adrenaline goes into the blood circulation and then signals the break down of glucogon in muscle and liver. The muscles have a sudden source of energy from glucose. GB has energy to run away and fortunately GB survives!

| Figure 3.10.

The hypothalamus sends an electrical signal to the adrenal gland under emergency conditions. The adrenal gland is stimulated to secrete adrenaline. Adrenaline stimulates the break-down of glycogen from muscle and liver. The break-down product of glycogen is glucose, an energy source for muscle. | 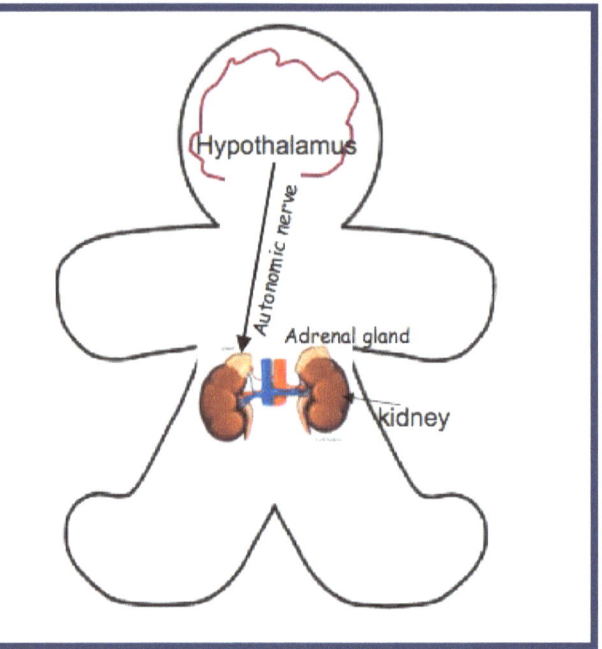 |

The direct link between a pathway and the nervous system is illustrated above for the production of adrenaline.

There is also much anecdotal evidence for the role of the brain in controlling metabolism. When people are sick we try to do something to "cheer them up", thinking that this will help the patient. People who develop new medicines notice that giving a patient a sugar pill instead of the drug often causes improvement. This is called the "placebo effect", and, and since interactions with other people is so important to us humans, the placebo effect is thought to be due to positive effects by the attention of the researcher on the patient.

Long-term stress, such as what someone may experience with an unsatisfactory personal or work situation (or students having too many exams!), causes the production of cortisol, which has major effects on metabolism. We will discuss more about cortisol in Chapter 6.

4. Power: Pathways that make ATP

4.1 The human body has a duel power system

In hybrid cars, such as a Prius™, power is supplied by two systems. For long-term travel, gasoline is used to move the pistons, which then causes the wheels to move. This process uses O_2 and an equation of the reaction of gasoline with oxygen, O_2, is the same as what occurs in metabolism:

$$C,H \text{ (gasoline in cars, food in people)} + O_2 \rightarrow CO_2 + H_2O + energy$$

The above reaction is said to be aerobic, meaning that it uses O_2.

The hybrid car has another power system; this system is electrical, powered by batteries that are charged when the car is moving. When the car is getting its energy from the electrical system, it is working anaerobically, meaning it is not using O_2.

The human body is much more complicated than a car, in part because we eat so many kinds of foods that are used as fuel. It is also much more efficient than a car; much of the power produced by a car is lost to friction. In this chapter we are going to tell how energy is produced in the cells of humans. We can think of this as how we produce power – the "power" being ATP, instead of the pistons that the car used.

Like a hybrid car, the human body has duel power systems. There is an anerobic system by which ATP is produced without using O_2. The anerobic pathway is called **glycolysis**. "Lysis" means "to break" and this pathway breaks sugars (6 C compounds) into 3 C compounds. The enzymes for this power system are located in the cytoplasm of the cell. Glycolysis is important in anerobic muscles. When you sprint or lift weights, you use this pathway. Glycolysis is also used when excess sugar is eaten. In this case sugar goes to 3 C in glycolysis, which then gets converted into fat.

The body, in addition, has an aerobic system. This power system resides in the mitochondria, and metabolic pathways in the mitochondria produce CO_2 and H_2O when the fuel reacts with O_2. This power system takes two C compounds and converts them to CO_2 in one pathway (called the **citric acid cycle**), H_2O is made from O_2 in a pathway called **oxidative phosphorylation**. The title of this latter pathway indicates that it requires O_2. The aerobic system produces most of the body's ATP. Without O_2 being supplied, death will occur rapidly, because most of tissues of the body rely on mitochondria to continually supply ATP.

4.2 Fuel for the engine: Starting materials for metabolism

Carbohydrates, fat and proteins are broken down into smaller components in the gastrointestinal tract.

When we think of sugar we usual think of table sugar. Table sugar molecules are composed of two different monosaccharides, fructose and glucose. Lactose is a sugar found in milk; it is composed of two sugars, galactose and glucose. Maltose is a disaccharide of two glucose molecules hooked together. Complex carbohydrates, such as flour and starch, get broken down into monosaccharides in the stomach and intestine.

33

Table 4.1 Disaccharides

Common disaccharide	Where we find it	Monosaccharide components
Sucrose	Table sugar	Fructose and glucose
lactose	Milk, dairy	Galactose and glucose
maltose	Barley and product of fermentation	Glucose and glucose

Monosaccharides sugar molecules enter the blood plasma from the intestinal tract. Some people have the inability to break down some of these compounds as their digestive systems lack a particular enzyme. In lactose intolerance, the enzyme to break lactose into glucose and galactose is missing or is defective. These people are advised to avoid milk products.

From the intestinal tract, the monosaccharide enters the portal vein system and gets transported to the liver.

Figure 4.1

Carbohydrates and amino acids from proteins are transported from the stomach and intestine via the portal vein. Blood exits the liver by the vena cava, which goes to the heart.   From the heart, the blood enters the general circulation.   The blood circulation insures that sugars and amino acids from digestion are first circulated through the liver. The liver can change these before they are put into circulation for use by all other tissues.

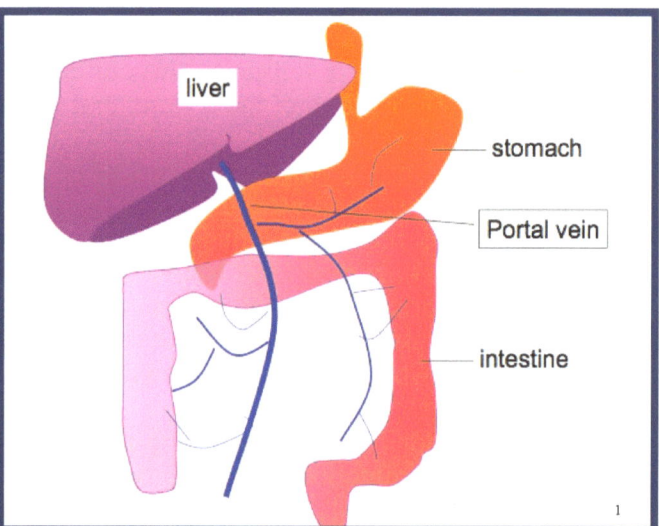

Just as carbohydrates are broken down to small units, proteins get digested to amino acids in the intestinal tract and are put into the portal vein.   This circulation ensures that the first organ that sees ingested carbohydrates and amino acids is the liver.   The liver can and does modify the molecules before putting the molecules into the blood of the vena cava, from where blood goes to the heart, and then is pumped throughout the body.

The digestion of fat and introduction of fat into the blood stream is different from carbohydrates and proteins and will be discussed in Chapter 7. The starting material for fat metabolism in the cell is a breakdown product of fat: it is fatty acid.

4.3 Overview of pathways that produce ATP

To summarize what we learned before, fats, proteins and carbohydrates are converted to CO_2 and H_2O and in this process ATP is formed. The word "pathway" is used to describe the sequence in the break-down of food. The word pathway is used to indicate that the compounds are not broken down willy-nilly, but are broken in a definite sequence, by enzymes. Enzymes are specialized proteins that are catalysts. A catalyst is a substance that makes a reaction go fast. Enzymes catalyze all chemical reactions in every pathway of the body. A pathway always involves the action of many enzymes.

Let's briefly go over what each pathway does. **Glycolysis** is the first pathway to metabolize sugar. This pathway, found in the cytoplasm breaks sugar into 3 C compounds, pyruvate and lactate. ATP is formed. In the mitochondria, the **pyruvate dehydrogenase** enzyme changes the 3 C compound is changed into 2 C compound (acetate in the form of acetyl CoA) and CO_2 is released. Extra H's are also formed, and temporarily stored in a compound called NADH

Fatty acids are changed into 2 C compound, acetyl CoA, and H's are transiently stored in NADH and FADH. (NADH and FADH are talked about in the next section). This pathway is called **β-oxidation**.

In metabolism food is converted into CO_2 and H_2O. The pathway that produces CO_2 is called the **citric acid cycle**. This pathway also transiently stores H in NADH and FADH. The pathway called **oxidative phosphorylation** takes H from NADH and FADH and adds it to O_2 that we get from breathing. This produces H_2O. In this pathway, many ATP are formed.

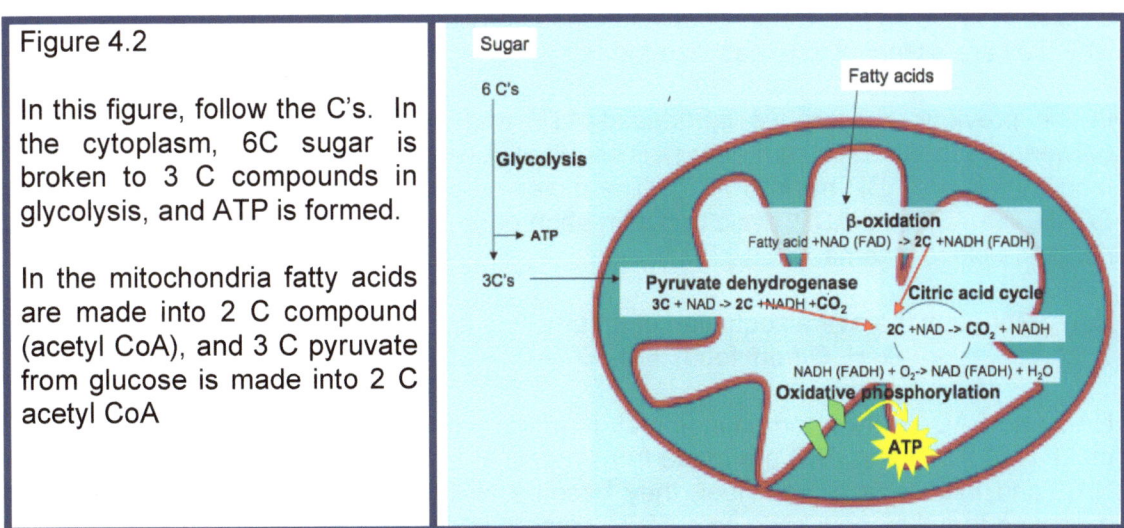

Figure 4.2

In this figure, follow the C's. In the cytoplasm, 6C sugar is broken to 3 C compounds in glycolysis, and ATP is formed.

In the mitochondria fatty acids are made into 2 C compound (acetyl CoA), and 3 C pyruvate from glucose is made into 2 C acetyl CoA

Figure 4.3	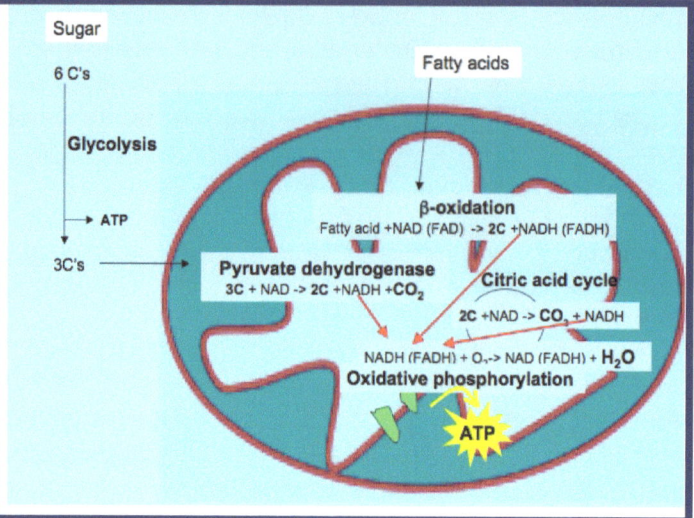
In this figure, look at the H's. H is gotten from fatty acids in β-oxidation, from 3C in pyruvate dehydrogenase, and from 2C in the citric acid cycle. The molecules that transiently store H's are NADH and FADH.	
The H's indirectly react with O_2 to form H_2O in oxidative phosphorylation. Many ATP molecules are formed.	

4.4 Four new compounds: NAD, NADH, FAD and FADH and importance of vitamins in metabolism

Before we describe how fuel makes ATP, we need to introduce a new concept in metabolism – the importance of vitamins. Two vitamins are described that required for cells to produce ATP. These vitamins are niacin (vitamin B_3) and flavin. We will describe why they are essential to metabolize food.
.
In the previous chapter we introduced ATP and ADP. These two molecules cycle between each other. When energy is required ATP goes to ADP. Then metabolism of food transforms ADP back to ATP. The molecule pairs, NAD and NADH, and FAD and FADH, like ATP and ADP, cycle between each other. Like ATP, they are inside of the cell, not in the blood plasma.

Remember that the overall equation of metabolism is:
$$(C, H, O \text{ from food}) + O_2 \rightarrow H_2O + CO_2 + \text{energy (as ATP)}$$

NAD and FAD are two compounds that, in effect, take H from food, and put it onto O_2 to make H_2O. NAD and FAD are made from vitamins, niacin and flavin, respectively. When NAD and FAD take H from fuel, they become NADH and FADH, the H in their name indicating that they now have an extra hydrogen, H. They indirectly add this H to O_2, and in so doing they return to being NAD and FAD, respectively.

Here is NAD (full name is nicotinamide adenine dinucleotide) and NADH (reduced nicotinamide adenine dinucleotide):

NAD and NADH are large molecules. The tail contains two ribose molecules (ribose is a 5C sugar), two phosphate groups (phosphate plus oxygen) and adenine. The adenine, ribose and two phosphates are identical to ADP, and this is an example of cellular economy. One molecule part is used for another. This tail helps to bind these molecules to specific enzymes. The business end is the nicotinamide end. This end gains hydrogen from food and loses hydrogen (H) to O_2 to form H_2O during metabolism.

Flavin adenine dinucleotide (FAD and FADH) is similar to NAD and NADH in that this pair also has a big tail. In the Figure below "R" represents the big tail.

The head part of the molecule is called flavin and it is shown above. It is where the action occurs – what changes during the chemical reaction. The big tail of FAD, like the tail of NAD, helps to hold these molecules in the proper location in the enzymes that use them.

Our bodies have enzymes that allow it to make ATP from smaller molecules, but we cannot synthesize (make) flavin or nicotinic acid; they are vitamins. A vitamin is a compound that is essential for our metabolism but which we cannot make from simple foods. From a biochemical point of view plants are more sophisticated than we are. Plants can make these compounds. We get them from the plants that we eat.

Part of NAD and NADH is nicotinamide, formed from nicotinic acid. "Nicotinic" sounds like something coming from cigarettes, but smoking does not give it to us. Grains have a high content of nicotinic acid. We also get it from meat, but the animals we eat in turn got it from plants. Another names for it is niacin and vitamin B_3. With a deficiency of the vitamin niacin in the diet, a disease called pellagra results. Symptoms of pellagra are skin lesions and general problems with metabolism. Nicotinic acid is used as part of NADH and NAD. It is also used in the synthesis of various compounds, seen in the next chapter. So, when vitamin B_3 is lacking, the enzymes that use NADH or NAD do not function and many organs are affected.

Niacin deficiency is very rare, as nicotinic acid is found in many foods. However, niacin deficiency is sometimes seen in alcoholics. These patients get most of their calories from alcohol and so their diets may be deficient in niacin. Alcoholism may also impair the absorption of niacin in the gut. Pellagra occurred in the American south during the first part of the 20th century. This was due to the prevalence of corn in the diet, lacking in niacin.

Flavin is also gotten from our foods and it is a vitamin. Flavin with a ribose sugar attached to it is called riboflavin. It is found in green plants, tomatoes and also in meat, eggs and milk. Riboflavin is used in many processes in the body, and deficiency in flavin, like a deficiency of niacin, causes general problems, including anemia. Children with riboflavin deficiency do not grow well.

Nicotinic acid and flavin are not stored in the body, and everyday they are excreted from the body in urine. Because they are lost each day, it is good to include fruits and vegetables in your diet every day! As a side point, flavin is fluorescent, and if you are taking vitamin supplements, you might notice that your urine has a fluorescent yellow-green color. Excess flavin is removed by the kidneys and gives a yellow-green color to urine.

4.5 Metabolism to make ATP

With this background, we now take a deep breath and go over the metabolic pathways that give energy. The pathways are summarized at the end of the chapter. Glucose breaks down to 3 carbon compounds. The 3 carbon compound then goes to 2 C, acetate (in the form of acetylCoA. Fatty acids break down to 2 C acetate also in the form of acetyl CoA. So the ending pathways are the same for glucose and fatty acids – both form acetylCoA. The acetate is broken to CO_2 and H_2O, forming ATP. Therefore, both glucose and fatty acids ultimately form CO_2 and H_2O.

4.5.1 Pathway 1. Glycolysis splits glucose to form two 3 C compounds; ATP formed

Glycolysis is the pathway that metabolizes sugars. Some common sugars are glucose, fructose and galactose. The figure represents a cell. All human cells have the glycolysis pathway in their cytoplasm. This pathway does not use O_2.

Figure 4.2	
Glycolysis. Each type of sugar has its own pump to get inside the cell. The pathway for glucose is shown. The first step in the pathway is to put a phosphate on glucose. The first step for galactose and fructose metabolism uses a different enzyme. After that the pathways are the same. The final products are pyruvate and lactate (3 carbon compounds)	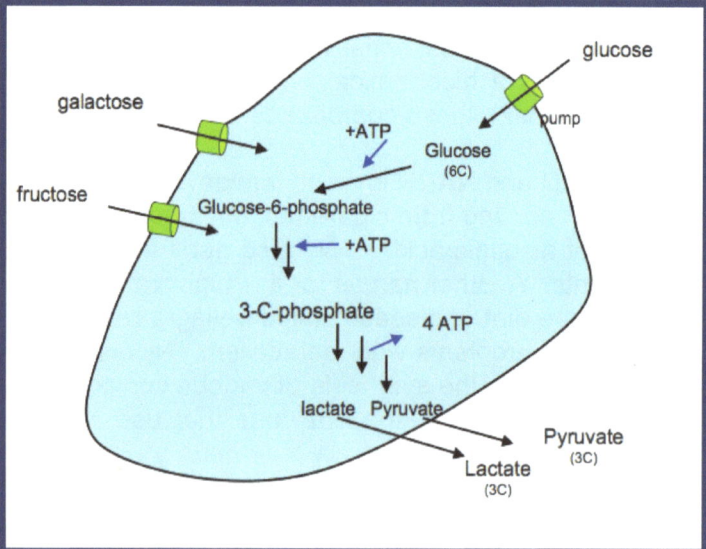

38

The initial step is to get glucose from blood into the cell. Various cells have different transporter molecules to take glucose from the blood. Glucose transporters in some tissues are sensitive to some hormones.

The hormone that has a major role in glucose transporters is insulin. Insulin is secreted by pancreas when glucose levels get high. When insulin is present, the transporters of fat and muscle become active and glucose goes inside these cells. The transporters in liver and brain cells are not sensitive to insulin. These tissues take in glucose whether insulin is present or not.

When glucose gets into the cell it gets phosphorylated. A phosphate gets put on to the 6th carbon position. The enzymes that do this are called glucokinase (in liver and pancreas) and hexokinase in other tissues. When two different enzymes catalyze the same reaction they are called isoenzymes. The picture of glucokinase was shown in Chapter 3, so you are already familiar with it. Glucokinase puts a phosphate group on glucose, to form glucose-6-phosphate:

Once the glucose has a phosphate on it, it is trapped inside the cell and the destiny of this molecule is to be changed somehow within the cell. Metabolites with phosphates on them do not circulate in the blood plasma. We already saw that with ATP, NADH and FADH.

Several things can happen to glucose-6-phosphate. It can be converted to the storage form of carbohydrates, glycogen. Alternatively, it can be used for synthesis of other molecules. Or, it can be broken to 3C compounds in reactions where ATP is made. This last pathway is glycolysis and is what we are interested in here.

In glycolysis, a series of enzyme-catalyzed reactions occur. All the intermediates have phosphate bound to them, and ultimately these phosphates get transferred to ADP to form ATP. Two ATP's are used to start the pathway, and 4 ATP's are formed. In the red blood cell, these extra two ATP's molecules are used to maintain the ion gradients in the cell.

The final step of glycolysis is the removal of phosphate from the intermediates to form lactate and pyruvate. Without phosphate, these compounds are free to leave the cell. This is what happens in the red blood cell, which has no mitochondria. Cells that have mitochondria can convert lactate and pyruvate to CO_2 and acetylCoA.

The products of glycolysis, **pyruvate** and **lactate,** have three C's. This is pyruvate:

The other product of glycolysis is lactate.

The difference between propionate and lactate is in the number of H's.

Here is where NADH comes into play. NADH adds H's to pyruvate; in losing H's it becomes NAD.

The glycolysis pathway is absolutely essential for human life. But only under some times, it becomes the major energy supply. During vigorous exercise, the supply of O_2 to muscle is not sufficient to supply the mitochondria so that mitochondria can keep up with production of ATP. Then glycolysis produces most of the ATP for the energy required for muscle contraction. This is called "anaerobic" exercise. (On an exercise bicycle, anaerobic exercise is when the muscles are rapidly contracting. Aerobic is a slower motion, that allows sufficient O_2 to be delivered to the mitochondria.)

In some cancer patients when the cancer is very advanced, high lactate in the blood indicates that glycolysis is producing much of the body's ATP. Glycolysis does not require O_2, and in large tumors, O_2 is not delivered to the center of the tumor, so glycolysis becomes predominant. But, like a hybrid car that cannot go for very long on the anaerobic electrical system, the human body cannot last very long solely on anaerobic metabolism of glycolysis. More ATP is required than what is supplied by glycolysis.

To summarize glycolysis: the final products of glycolysis are lactate/pyruvate and ATP. For each glucose molecule that is metabolized to two pyruvate or lactate molecules, two ATP molecules are formed.

4.5.2 Pathway 2. Pyruvate dehydrogenase splits three C into two C plus CO_2; NADH formed

Pyruvate has 3C's and it comes from glucose, via glycolysis and it is also a product of some amino acids. First, pyruvate enters the mitochondria. Then the pyruvate dehydrogenase[1] enzyme chops pyruvate into acetate and CO_2. In doing this, it converts an ADP molecule into ATP.

This is the first time where we see the production of CO_2, the final product of metabolism. CO_2 goes into the blood stream and it leaves the body in the lungs. The other two products of the pyruvate dehydrogenase reaction are acetate and NADH. Pyruvate dehydrogenase ties up acetic acid with coenzyme A, abbreviated CoA. This is acetyl CoA:

The CoA tail prevents acetate from leaving the mitochondrion, just as phosphate prevents glucose-6-phosphate and other intermediates of glycolysis from leaving cells. The final products of pyruvate dehydrogenase are ATP, NADH, acetylCoA and CO_2. You notice that we have gotten energy, ATP, from the action of the pyruvate dehydrogenase enzyme.

---

[1] The names of many enzymes end in "-ase". In contrast, note on Table 4.1 that sugar molecules end in "-ose."

4.5.3. Pathway 3. β-oxidation breaks fatty acid to 2 C; FADH and NADH formed

The break-down of fat into CO_2, yields many calories in the form of ATP. The starting material in fat metabolism is a fatty acid, shown here:

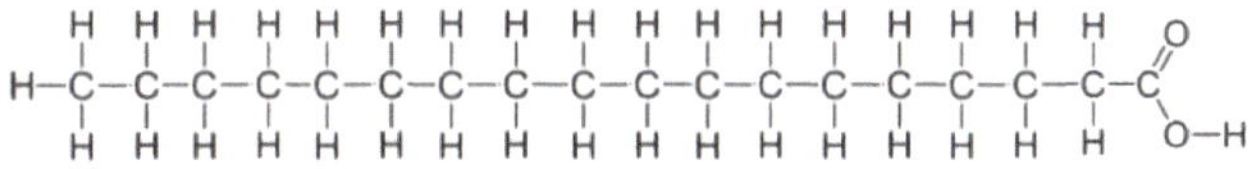

First, a CoA is added by an enzyme to keep the fatty acid inside the cell:

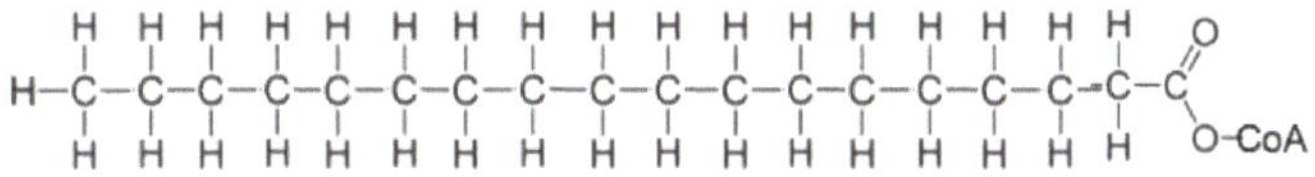

Then an O atom is placed at the third C. In chemistry the first C from the carboxy end is called the α (alpha) C and the second one is called the β (beta) C. Hence, this pathway is called β oxidation.

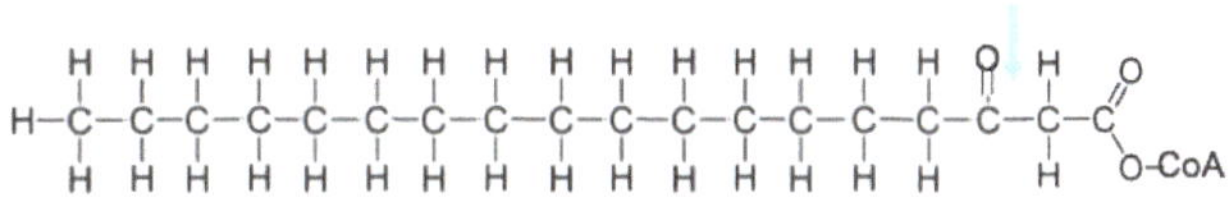

In putting the O onto the fatty acid, NAD goes to NADH and FAD (flavin) goes to FADH.

Next, the fatty acid splits at the place indicated by the blue arrow. The two products are acyl CoA and acetylCoA. The two products have similar sounding names! Acetyl CoA means a two C unit; it is a derivative of acetate. Acyl is a generic name for any fatty acid group, irrespective of the number of C's.

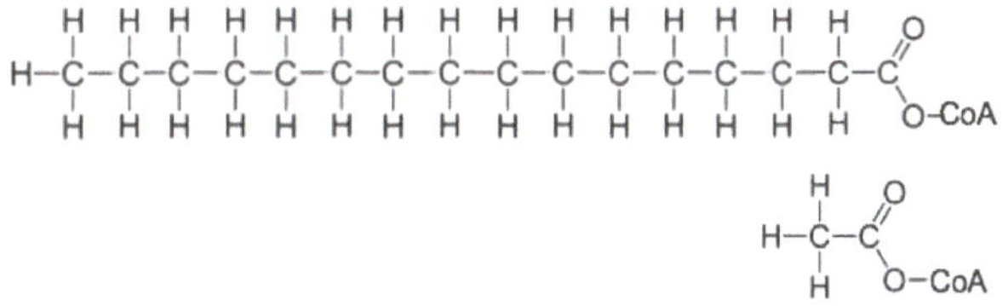

You see that you have gotten acetylCoA and a fatty acid CoA that is two C's shorter than the starting acid. Then the process starts over. The 16 C fatty acid is chopped to become 14 C plus acetyl CoA, each time producing NADH and FADH. Then again and again, to make 12 C, then 10 C, then 8 C and so on until finally all the fatty acid is chopped down to acetyl CoA.

The final products of β-oxidation are acetyl CoA, NADH and FADH.

4.5.4 Pathway 4. Citric acid cycle takes two C (acetyl CoA) to CO_2; NADH and FADH formed

Acetyl-CoA is formed from the breakdown of fat (via β-oxidation) and of sugar (via glycolysis and pyruvate dehydrogenase). Acetyl-CoA is oxidized by O_2 to CO_2 in a series of steps in the mitochondria. This pathway is called the **citric acid cycle.** It is called a cycle because the molecules that are involved in the pathway regenerate themselves, and the word citric refers to one of compounds in the cycle. We will also mention the citric acid cycle later when protein use as food is discussed. Acetyl-CoA combines with a 4 C compound. Then, in a series of steps, those two C's that came from acetate get chopped off to form CO_2, and the 4 C compound is regenerated.

41

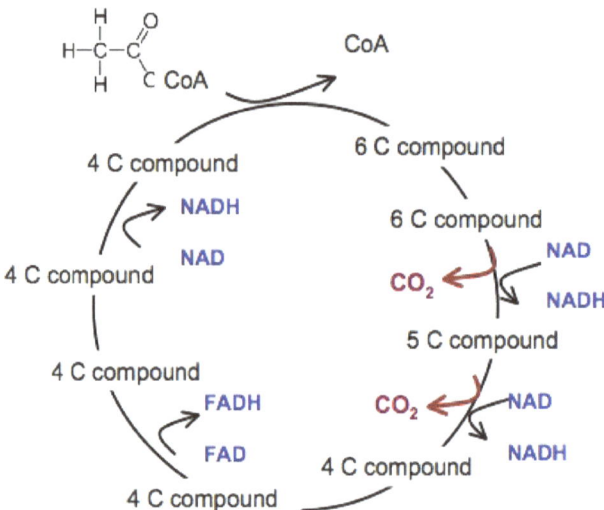

Every acetyl group gets converted to two CO_2 molecules. Once acetyl gets into the pathway, it is the end of it in the body. The CO_2 produced goes into blood, the blood transports it to the lungs, and from the lungs it is exhaled to the atmosphere. To convert acetyl to CO_2, three NAD's and one FAD are reduced to NADH and FADH, respectively.

The final products of the citric acid cycle are CO_2, NADH and FADH.

4.5.5 Pathway 5. Oxidative phosphorylation uses O_2 to make H_2O; NADH and FADH transformed back to NAD and FAD with the formation of ATP

Oxidative phosphorylation is the powerhouse ATP producing pathway of the body. Oxidative phosphorylation is the pathway where FADH and NADH from pyruvate dehydrogenase, β-oxidation and the citric acid cycle ultimately react with O_2 to produce H_2O, the other final product of metabolism. In so doing, FADH and NADH are converted back to FAD and NAD, respectively. While this is happening, ADP is phosphorylated to form ATP.

The proteins that catalyze oxidative phosphorylation are embedded in the inner membrane of the mitochondria. Many of the proteins that carry out these reactions are colored like hemoglobin, the protein that makes blood red.

| Figure 4.3.

Enzymes in the membrane of mitochondria use NADH to add an H to O_2 This produces H_2O and NAD. In this process a phosphate is added to ADP to make ATP. | |

42

Electrons are transferred between these proteins in the membrane of mitochondria. NADH goes back to NAD and O_2 goes to H_2O. During these processes, ATP is made from ADP. For each NADH converted back to NAD, 3 ATP's are formed. For FADH going to FAD, two ATP's are formed. You can see why the mitochondria are the cell's power house.

The pathways used at a given time depend whether we are using fat or sugar for energy. There is one pathway, glycolysis, and one single step, pyruvate dehydrogenase, for sugar metabolism. There is another pathway, β-oxidation, for fat. These pathways converge since the C product of both sugar and fat is acetate, a 2C compound. Acetate is bound in a compound called acetyl CoA. Acetate is degraded to CO_2 in the citric acid cycle (pathway 4). The citric acid cycle produces NADH, which is described below. NADH reacts with O_2 in a series of reactions to form ATP.

4.6 Road map of pathways

Figures 4.4 and 4.5 summarize the pathways for glucose (sugar) and fat metabolism. Note that CO_2 and H_2O are the final products of metabolism of both fat and carbohydrates. The metabolism of both leads to ATP production.

Proteins also give us energy. Proteins are broken down to amino acids in the intestine. Like fat and carbohydrates, amino acids are metabolized to form CO_2 and H_2O, thereby producing ATP. Some amino acids are metabolized using the pathways for glucose; some are metabolized like fatty acids.

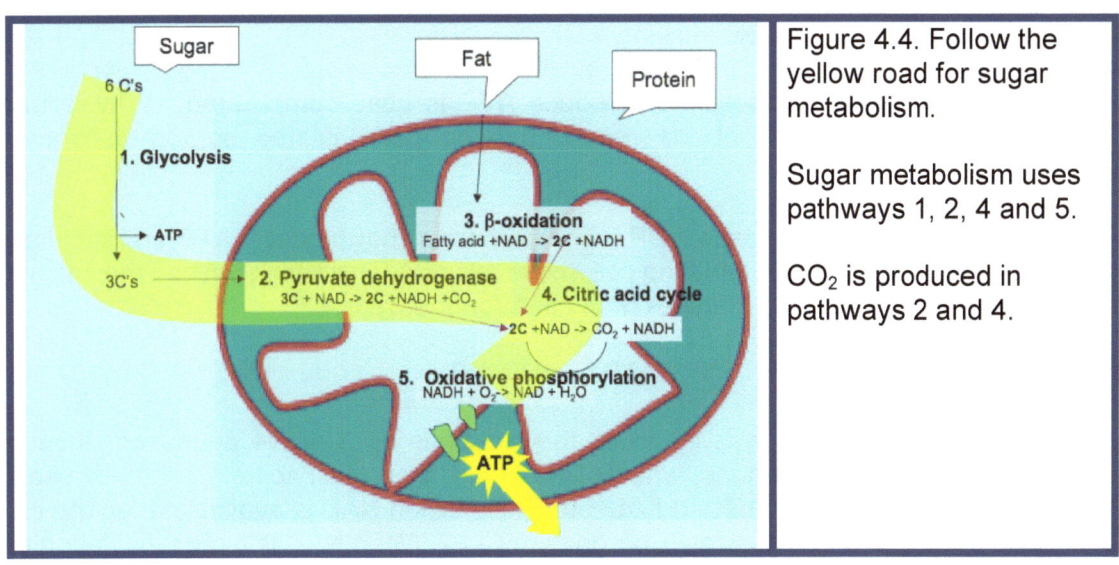

Figure 4.4. Follow the yellow road for sugar metabolism.

Sugar metabolism uses pathways 1, 2, 4 and 5.

CO_2 is produced in pathways 2 and 4.

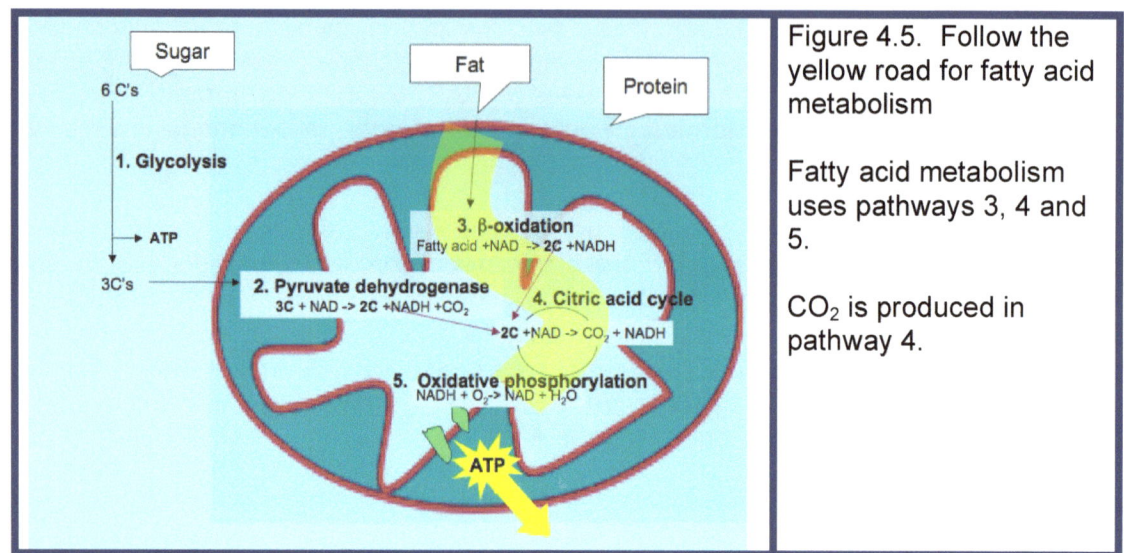

Figure 4.5. Follow the yellow road for fatty acid metabolism

Fatty acid metabolism uses pathways 3, 4 and 5.

CO_2 is produced in pathway 4.

4.7 When do these pathways operate? How is the production of ATP regulated?

The pathways are complex, but in a way they are quite simple. The simple version is that six C sugars goes to three C molecules, which then gets converted to two C's. Fatty acids get converted to two C's. The two C molecule, coming either from glucose or fat, goes to CO_2. The side products of these reactions, FADH and NADH, put an H on O_2 to produce H_2O, this process coincides with making ATP.

At a deeper level the metabolism to produce ATP is quite complicated. Why is that? Probably, it is because all of the reactions must be regulated so that balance is maintained.

The major regulating molecule is ADP. The pathways that produce ATP are stimulated when the cell needs ATP. In a resting cell, the levels of ATP are high. When the cell uses energy, ATP goes to ADP, because ATP is used for energy.

$$ATP \rightarrow ADP + P$$

At high ATP, oxidation by O_2 is inhibited: the reactions of oxidative phosphorylation are not going on. On the other hand, when ADP is high, then mitochondria suddenly use O_2 and they oxidize NADH to NAD and FADH to FAD. When NAD is available, then the citric acid cycle goes into gear and acetylCoA goes to CO_2. When NAD is high, β-oxidation can occur and fatty acids get broken down. When NAD is high, pyruvate dehydrogenase is activated, so that propionylCoA goes to acetylCoA and CO_2.

So these three pathways all go fast when ADP is high, indicating the cell needs ATP. Oxidative phosphorylation, citric acid cycle, β–oxidation and pyruvate dehydogenase pathways slow down when ATP is high. All of these mitochondrial pathways depend upon O_2 to keep NAD and FAD ready to accept H atoms.

4.8 Hormones regulate metabolism

When you look at the pathways, you can see another question. You notice that acetylCoA can come from fat or from glucose. How does the cell "know" which food source to use? The answer is easy for the brain. The blood brain barrier does not allow fat to go into the brain. So the brain uses glucose under usual conditions (and keto-acids coming from fat during starvation). For other tissues the major regulation is by the hormone insulin. When blood sugar is high, the pancreas produces insulin. Insulin prevents the breakdown of fat to fatty acid, and therefore β-oxidation does not occur. Insulin stimulates glycolysis and pyruvate dehydrogenase. Therefore the acetylCoA used in the citric acid cycle will be obtained from glucose. Excess acetylCoA from glucose is made into fat (Chapter 6). Insulin also stimulates the production of fat from glucose.

When a person does not have sugar in the blood, insulin is low. Low insulin stimulates the release of fatty acids from adipose.

We will discuss how insulin works on important enzymes of metabolism in Chapter 11.

Glycolysis is hormonally regulated indirectly by insulin, but it also sensitive to low energy levels, i.e., low ATP, in the cell. Unlike oxidative phosphorylation, which is stimulated by ADP, glycolyis is stimulated by AMP, which stands for adenosine monophosphate. AMP is made from ADP, catalyzed by an enzyme called myokinase. The reaction is:

$$2ADP \rightarrow ATP + AMP$$

When ADP is high, this reaction takes a phosphate from one ADP on another one and makes ATP, which can then be used for energy by the cell. The remainder AMP stimulates glycolysis, and by this means more ATP is supplied.

4.9 Insulin regulates the fuel sources

The metabolism of carbohydrates and fat gives us ATP. The figure below illustrates how the pathways are regulated by one hormone, insulin, and by the energy requirement of the cell.

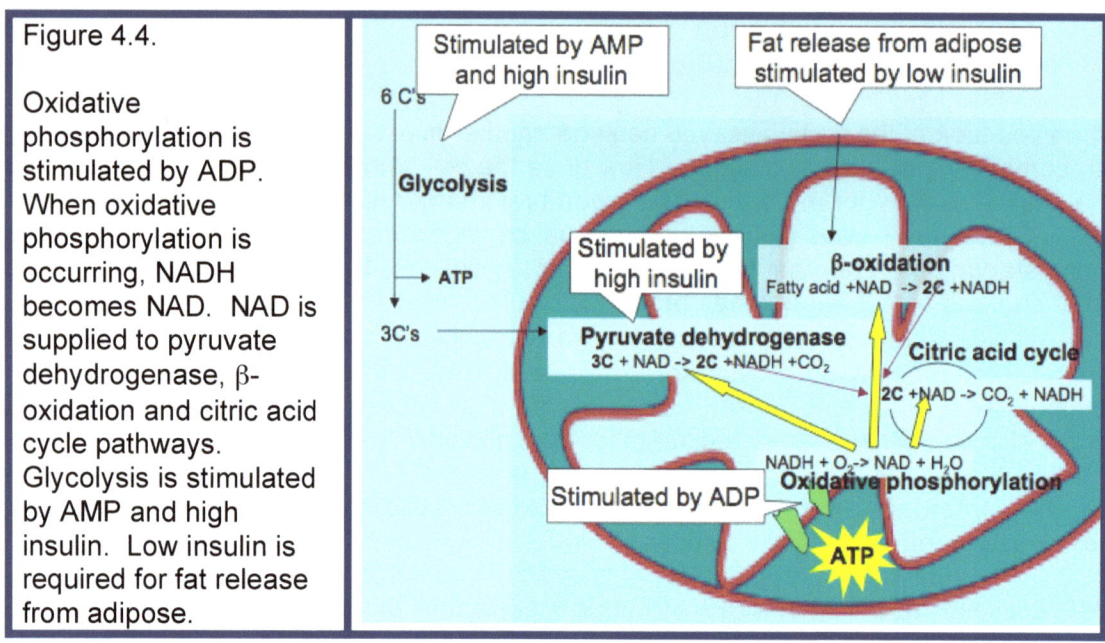

Figure 4.4.

Oxidative phosphorylation is stimulated by ADP. When oxidative phosphorylation is occurring, NADH becomes NAD. NAD is supplied to pyruvate dehydrogenase, β-oxidation and citric acid cycle pathways. Glycolysis is stimulated by AMP and high insulin. Low insulin is required for fat release from adipose.

4.10 Long term regulation: lactate threshold

In exercise, the point where lactate is produced is called the lactate threshold. This occurs where O_2 supply does not keep up with the requirement for ATP, and is unable to remove the lactate produced from glycolysis. A trained athlete will be able exercise for a longer period compared to a "couch potato" before lactate builds up. The training program of an athlete increases the number of mitochondria in the muscle, the amount of capillaries and the power of the heart, so that O_2 can be delivered faster. Changing the level of the enzymes is a long-term regulation of metabolism.

Thyroid hormone also controls metabolism. People who have low thyroid have low metabolism, meaning that these pathways are going slowly. With excess thyroid, these pathways run in full gear. But, thyroid hormone does not directly act on the enzymes of mitochondria or glycolysis. It uses another form of regulation that is not fully understood.

4.11 Cases

4.11.1 Diseases where ATP levels are too low in red blood cells

Here are descriptions of two diseases that involves glycolysis and affects red blood cells (RBCs). These diseases are both described as being hemolytic anemia. Hemolytic means that the RBC's break down too soon. ("Hemo" refers to blood and "lytic" comes from the word lysis, to break apart). A normal RBC lasts in the blood for about 120 days. If the RBC is defective for some reason, the RBC is taken out of circulation sooner than that, and the patient will have fewer RBCs. The patient will have anemia – not enough RBCs. In the following cases patients have similar symptoms, but the reasons for the hemolytic anemia are different.

Case 1: Hemolytic anemia in hospital patients. (Travis, S. F. et al, New England J. Med. 285, 763-768 (1971)

46

A group of 8 patients were recovering in the hospital following gastrointestinal surgery. They were in the hospital for 3 to 4 weeks, during which time they were given nutrition through a catheter in the subclavian vein. The nutrition included amino acids, glucose and vitamins.

The hematocrit and hemoglobin was low (8-10 g/dl; normal 12-15 g/dl) for these patients. These two values showed the doctors that the patient had lower than normal amount of red blood cells (RBC's) The researchers took blood from the patients and examined the red blood cells. They lyzed the cells to release the enzymes contained in the cells and to examine the levels of metabolites. They found that the enzymes in the RBC's were normal, but the level of ATP was low. They also found that phosphate levels were low.

Diagnosis, treatment and discussion: In this case, the patients suffered from a nutritional lack of phosphate. With a low level of phosphate, the conversion of ADP to ATP was slow. If ATP is not regenerated fast enough, ATP levels will decrease. ATP is constantly be used to maintain the salt levels in RBC's. Without the proper salt levels, RBC's will be unstable.

These patients were treated by including phosphate in their intravenous (IV) nutrition. This kind of hemolytic anemia caused by phosphate deficiency is no longer seen in hospital patients with long-term IV nutrition because, after this paper was published, phosphate is included in the intravenous fluid.

Case 2. Hemolytic anemia in a boy. (Br. J. Hematol. 132, 523-9, 2008, Noel N., Flanagan, JM et al)

This patient was the only son of a healthy couple from Barcelona. Pregnancy was normal, but after delivery the baby showed severe anemia (Hb 7.3 g/dl; normal 10-12) and jaundice. Jaundice occurs because there is an elevated amount of bilirubin, a break-down product of hemoglobin. The anemia recovered without blood transfusion. Red blood cell morphology appeared normal under a microscopy. At 2 years of age, the patient was hospitalized due to severe anemia (Hb 6.6 g/dl) and jaundice for which he received exchange transfusion and antibiotics. The diagnosis of a deficiency in an enzyme of glycolysis was established at the age of 3 years during a hemolytic crisis. Blood sample was taken from the boy and tests for enzyme activities was undertaken. After examining the enzymes in the RBC's, diagnosis was made. This patient has phosphoglycerate kinase deficiency.

Diagnosis, treatment and discussion: This patient has a defect in an enzyme that takes a phosphate from an intermediate of glycolysis and puts it on ATP. Because this enzyme was defective, the ATP levels in the RBC's are low, because glycolysis cannot go fast enough to keep the ATP high. Blood transfusion will alleviate the anemia. Since glycolysis is required for all cells, and nerve cells use glucose, not fat, for metabolism, they are also affected. The boy continued to be ill. At 7 years of age the hemolytic crises were associated with a progressive neurological impairment leading to mental retardation

The above two cases illustrate two examples of metabolic diseases. The first is a nutritional disease. The second is a genetic disease that runs in families. Both affect glycolysis; in both cases glycolysis becomes slower than it should be to keep ATP levels high to maintain the salt levels. In both cases the hematocrit (number of red blood cells in the blood) and hemoglobin is low because the RBC's are degrading too fast. These diseases particularly affect RBC's because RBC's do not have mitochondria, which supply most cells with most of their ATP. Note that at longer times, the brain of the boy was affected. Glycolysis is needed for brain function.

4.11.2 Case where mitochondria do not produce enough ATP

The case below shows disturbed metabolism in mitochondria.

> **Case 3:   Coma in a family on a holiday trip** (Adapted from: http://www.cdc.gov/mmwr/preview/mmwrhtml/mm5402a2.htm)
>
> Family of four (husband, wife and two children) went on an annual Christmas vacation to their cabin in the north woods. An oil furnace heated the cabin. After unwrapping their presents on Christmas eve, the family went to bed.
>
> The husband awoke at 2:30 AM feeling nauseous and confused. He was unable to wake his wife or his children. He called 911.
>
> **Diagnosis, treatment and discussion:** The emergency response team gave the family members oxygen and opened the windows of the cabin. All family members responded by becoming alert. They had no long-term effects. The diagnosis was CO (carbon monoxide) intoxication, due to faulty ventilation of the oil furnace.
>
> CO is deadly because CO replaces O_2 in hemoglobin, and consequently there is not enough O_2 to maintain oxidative phosphorylation. CO also inhibits the last enzyme in oxidative phosphorylation. For these two reasons, oxidative phosphorylation is slowed. Not enough ATP is produced by the mitochondria to maintain functions of the cell. Without a constant supply of ATP in the brain, death occurs.

4.12 "Cheat sheet" of pathways

This has been an arduous chapter. If you take a deep breath, and look out the window, you might see trees, grass, birds, dogs and people. All of these multicelled organisms use the pathways that have been described here. So, although this chapter is hard, you have learned a lot of biology in one fell swoop. In case of plants, metabolism is even more complicated than for human metabolism, because plants have more metabolic pathways than we. They also carry out photosynthesis and make all the amino acids that they need.

To help you keep the pathways straight, the pathways that produce ATP are listed in Table 4.2.

Table 4.2. Pathways for energy production

	Pathway	Location	Starting compound and its fate	Ending compound	Energy compound
1	Glycolysis	Cytoplasm Does not require O_2	**Glucose** (6 C's) gets converted to 3 C (pyruvate and lactate).	Pyruvate, lactate (3C)	Net **2 ATP's formed**
2	Pyruvate dehydrogenase	mitochondria	**Pyruvate** (3 C's) gets converted to 2C's (acetyl CoA) and CO_2.	Acetate (2C as acetyl CoA)	NADH produced from NAD; One ATP molecule formed
3	β-oxidation of fatty acids	mitochondria	**Fatty acids** broken to 2 C units (acetyl CoA)	Acetate (2C as acetyl CoA)	NADH produced from NAD; FADH produced from FAD
4	Citric acid cycle	mitochondria	**Acetyl CoA** gets converted to CO_2	CO_2	NADH produced from NAD; FADH produced from FAD
5	Oxidative phosphorylation *Powerhouse*	mitochondria	NADH goes to NAD; FADH goes to FAD; O_2 goes to H_2O.	H_2O	NADH to NAD, 3 ATP formed. FADH to FAD, 2 ATP formed.

5. Storage and retrieval from glycogen: Metabolism during short term fasting

5.1 Storage form of carbohydrates is glycogen; Glycogen is fuel for quick energy

The whole of metabolism is this:
$$C,H,O \text{ (food)} + O_2 \rightarrow CO_2 + H_2O + \textit{energy}$$
This is the overall reaction that gives us ATP, as we outlined in the previous chapter. We emphasized that this reaction must occur at all times. We get O_2 from breathing, and we must breathe at all times. The other part of metabolism is C, H and O, which represent the major elements in food.

Luckily for us, our bodies store food, so we do not have to be eating all the time. Without our bodies storing food, civilization would cease because we would have no time for education, music, art, work or hanging out with friends.

We already know that the three forms of food are carbohydrates, proteins and fat – and these forms of food are also stored for fuel. But we do not store the same molecules that we eat. They must be processed to be suitable for storage. And there must be a way to retrieve the stored molecules when the body needs energy from the stored molecules.

The various types of stored fuel are retrieved in different ways and at different times. Figure 1 shows what metabolites are supplying to GB after eating, and then during fasting and starvation.

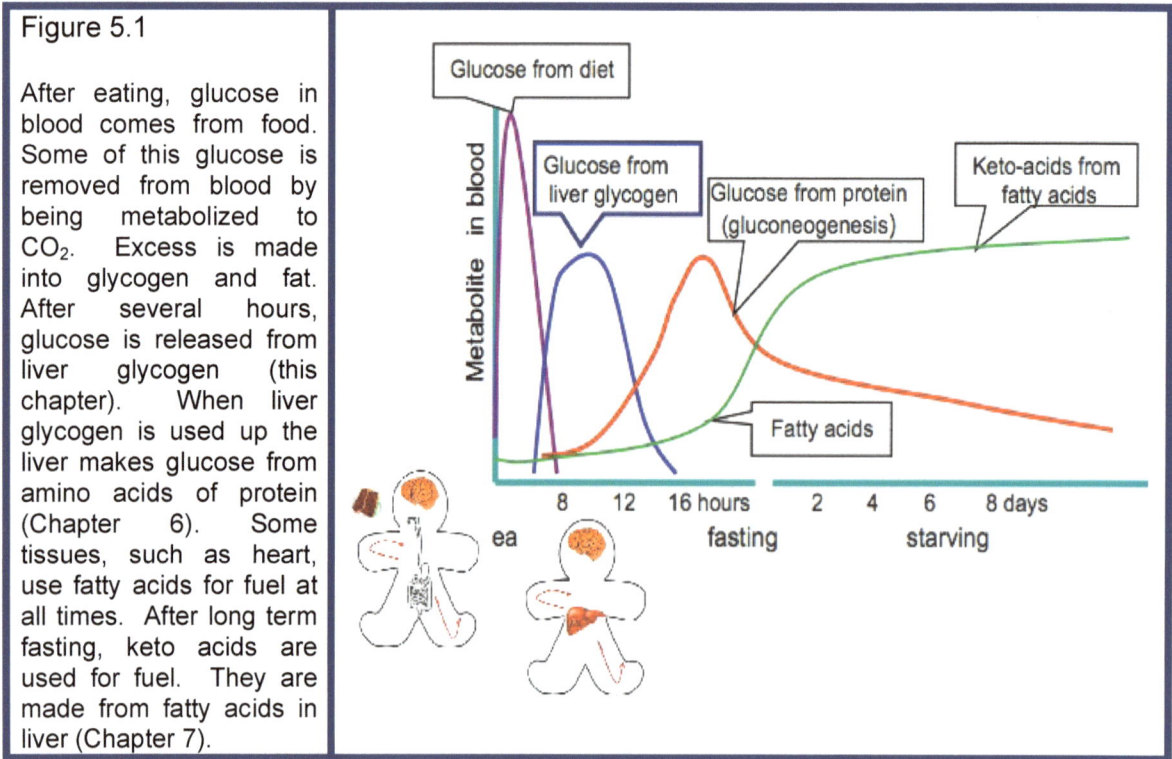

Figure 5.1

After eating, glucose in blood comes from food. Some of this glucose is removed from blood by being metabolized to CO_2. Excess is made into glycogen and fat. After several hours, glucose is released from liver glycogen (this chapter). When liver glycogen is used up the liver makes glucose from amino acids of protein (Chapter 6). Some tissues, such as heart, use fatty acids for fuel at all times. After long term fasting, keto acids are used for fuel. They are made from fatty acids in liver (Chapter 7).

This chapter deals with the storage and retrieval of fuel from carbohydrates. The next two chapters discuss protein and fat, respectively.

Carbohydrate is stored as glycogen. We are starting with glycogen because we are thinking of our patient, GB, and what happens after he eats. Glycogen is mobilized for energy after a short term fast. Glycogen is made from glucose and in the liver it breaks back down into glucose. This glucose goes into the blood stream and supplies fuel for the brain. In other tissues, glycogen breaks down into glucose-1-phosphate, and the particular tissue uses this for its own fuel. The two organs that have large glycogen stores are liver and muscle.

5.2 Glycogen in liver and muscle

All tissues store glycogen. But because so much of our overall metabolism occurs in liver and muscle, these tissues are emphasized. Here is the overview of the storage and release of fuel from these two tissues:

> **Liver** is the unselfish "good-guy" of metabolism. Liver takes sugar from the blood stream and makes it into glycogen after eating. When glucose in the blood gets low, glycogen stored in the liver is broken down to glucose. This glucose goes out from liver into the blood stream. The brain (and other tissues) picks up this glucose from the blood and uses it for energy. The source of fuel from liver glycogen for the brain is especially important for short term fasting. Short-term is, say, less than about 12 hours after eating.

> **Muscle** uses both fat and glucose for energy, but fast, white muscles, used for sudden motion, primarily use mostly glycogen as a fuel. Muscle stores glycogen, and muscle's stored glycogen gets broken down into glucose-6-phosphate. The glucose that comes from muscle glycogen never leaves the muscle cells, and instead, glucose 6-phosphate gets converted to 3 C compound (pyruvate and lactate). Consequently, the muscle uses its glycogen for itself. Muscle is "selfish"– it does not directly share glucose from its stored glycogen with other organs.

5.3 Hormones regulate the use of glycogen

The use of glycogen is different in the liver and in muscle. Glycogen storage and release in both tissues are hormonally controlled.

One player is **insulin**, which was introduced in the last chapter. Three other hormonal players are **epinephrine**, **glucogon and cortisol**. Insulin stimulates the storage of fuel; Epinephrine, glucogon and cortisol stimulate the release of fuel from storage in the tissue. "Glucogon" sounds a lot like "glycogen" but we remember that:

> *glucogon* is a hormone
> and
> *glycogen* is the storage form of sugar

Both glucogon and insulin are made in the pancreas. The pancreas is an organ that lies behind the stomach and under the liver, and it makes both endocrine and exocrine hormones and enzymes. Glucogon and insulin are **endocrine** hormones; the pancreas secretes them into blood plasma, not the digestive tract. Pancreas also excretes enzymes that are used to break down food in the digestive tract; these enzymes are considered exocrine enzymes.

Glucogon and insulin are both made of amino acids, so they are classified as polypeptides (in effect they are miniature proteins). The pancreas contains a specialized substructure, picturesquely called "Islets of Langerhans". One type of cell within the islets is the α (alpha) cell. α cells secrete glucogon. Another type of cell is the β (beta) cell. β cells secrete insulin. At "normal" glucose levels, a low level of insulin is secreted but after a high carbohydrate and protein meal glucose and amino acid levels in the blood go up. The β cells respond to high glucose by secreting insulin into the blood. Insulin acts on many tissues, and its action is to reduce glucose levels in the blood. Without eating, glucose levels decrease more and more in the blood. Then the hormone glucogon comes into play. Its function is to stimulate the release of glucose from stored glycogen, thereby increasing glucose levels in the blood.[2]

Two other hormones act to increase blood glucose levels. Both are made in the adrenal cortex, a gland that is above the kidneys. Epinephrine is derived from an amino acid, and it is a hormone that elicits a short-term release of glucose from stores.[34] Cortisol is the third hormone; it is produced in the cortex of the kidneys. Cortisol is derived from cholesterol. It acts to stimulate the making of glucose from protein. We will discuss the role of cortisol in maintaining glucose levels the next chapter.

5.4 Storage of carbohydrates after eating

5.4.1 Liver

In the previous chapter we showed what happens to glucose when ATP is required: glucose gets transformed to a 3 C compound with the production of ATP by glycolysis. Then it gets chopped to 2 C, which goes to CO_2 in the mitochondria. In doing this, mitochondria consume O_2 and produce ATP.

Now we look at what happens when the liver cell has more glucose than needed to make ATP for its energy needs. After a high carbohydrate meal, glucose in the blood plasma is high. High glucose stimulates the pancreatic β-cell to secrete insulin. Insulin stimulates glycogen synthesis. Glycogen does not accumulate indefinitely, however. Unlike fat where we can store more and more (getting fatter and fatter), when the glycogen store is

---

[2] There are two other types of cells in the Islets of Langerhans. The d cells secrete somatostatin and the PP cells secrete pancreatic polypeptide. These hormones serve to regulate insulin and glucogon. So we have hormones regulating other hormones! But for the level of discussion here, we will not consider the action of somatostatin and pancreatic polypeptide.

[3] Another name for epinephrine is adrenaline.

[4] Epinephrine controls blood flow and makes the heart beat faster. There is a related compound called norepinephrine that also plays a role. We are interested in metabolism here, but only point out that the effects of hormones are more complex than what we describe.

filled, no more goes in. When liver is "full" of glycogen, glycogen accounts for about 10 % of the weight of the liver. [5] After the glycogen store is filled, excess sugar gets transformed to 3 C's (lactate and pyruvate), then to 2 C's (acetyl group in acetylCoA) and then made into fat.

After eating, when glucose in the blood is high, insulin is secreted. So insulin in blood goes high while glucogon secretion goes down. Consequently, after eating carbohydrate, the hormone ratio of insulin to glucogon (I/G) is high. This hormone set stimulates the storage of glycogen in the liver and the transformation of excess glucose into fat. Figure 5.2 diagrams this.

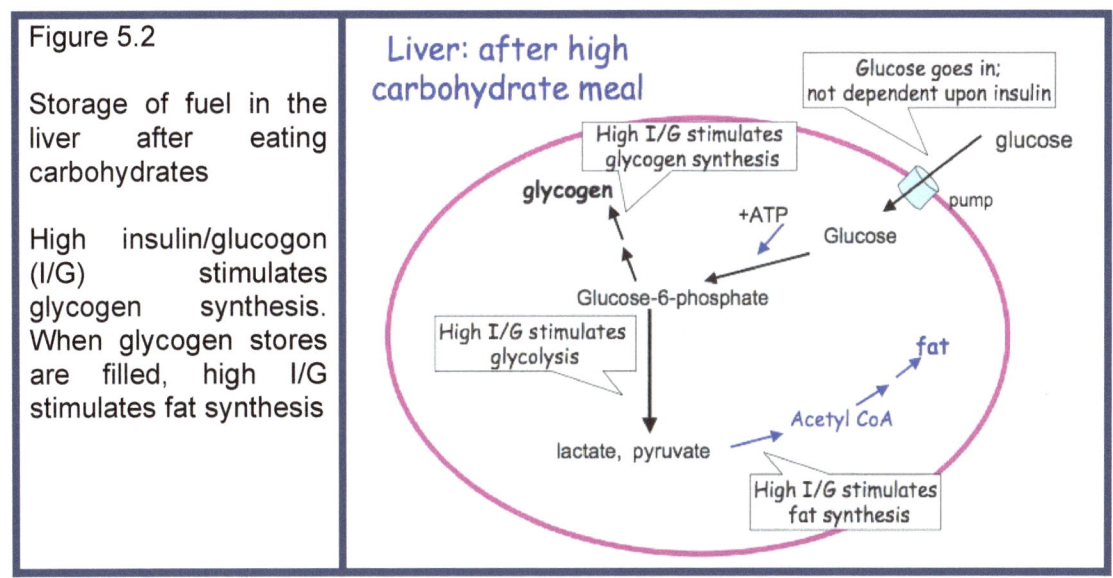

Figure 5.2

Storage of fuel in the liver after eating carbohydrates

High insulin/glucogon (I/G) stimulates glycogen synthesis. When glycogen stores are filled, high I/G stimulates fat synthesis

5.4.2 Muscle

Muscle, like liver, takes in glucose to make glycogen after a high carbohydrate meal, when I/G is high. Glucose is also taken into the muscle during exercise, even when insulin is low. These processes are diagramed in Figure 5.3.

---

[5] You might have noticed that in the morning your abdomen feels flatter than at night. This is because the stored glycogen in the liver has been used up overnight.

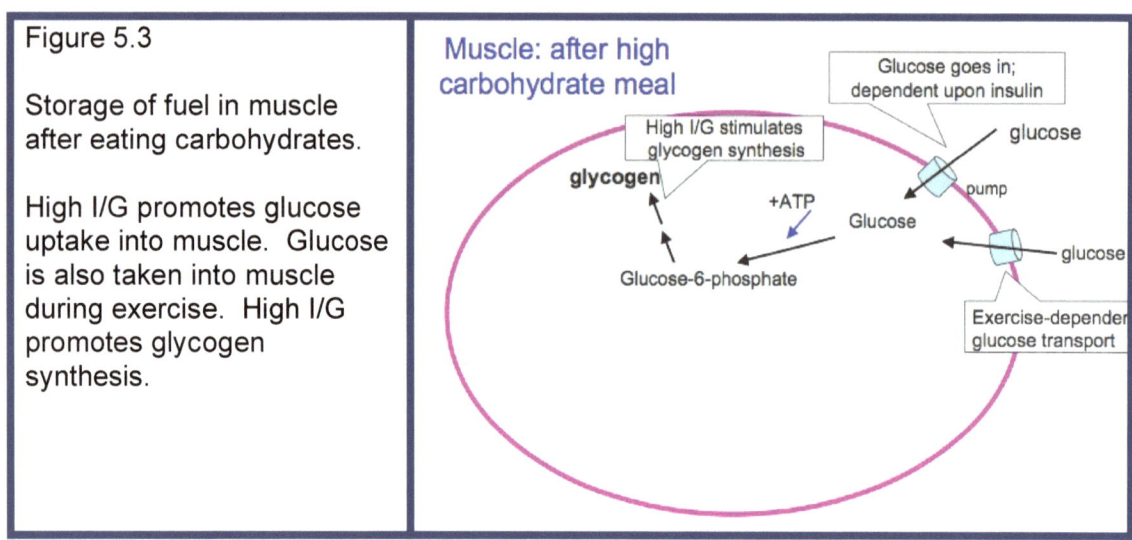

Figure 5.3

Storage of fuel in muscle after eating carbohydrates.

High I/G promotes glucose uptake into muscle. Glucose is also taken into muscle during exercise. High I/G promotes glycogen synthesis.

5.5 How glucose is released from glycogen

5.5.1 Liver – the good guy

We learned in Chapter 4 that fat gets broken down into acetyl CoA, which gets oxidized to CO_2 in the citric acid cycle. The acetyl group has two Cs, and consequently two CO_2 molecules are formed from it. So fatty acids are not converted into glucose – they get broken to CO_2; CO_2 is lost in breathing. The brain needs glucose for metabolism. The brain is selective in what it takes from the blood. The brain is protected by what is called the "blood-brain barrier". The capillaries in the brain form a barrier that prevents the brain from taking fatty acids in the blood.

So, there needs to be a source for glucose and the source of glucose for the brain is the liver. Under "short-term" fasting conditions, glycogen in the liver gets degraded back to glucose. Hormones control the breakdown of glycogen to form glucose-6-phosphate. When glucose is low, insulin goes down, and glucogon goes up. This is the trigger for the enzymes that break down glycogen to act.

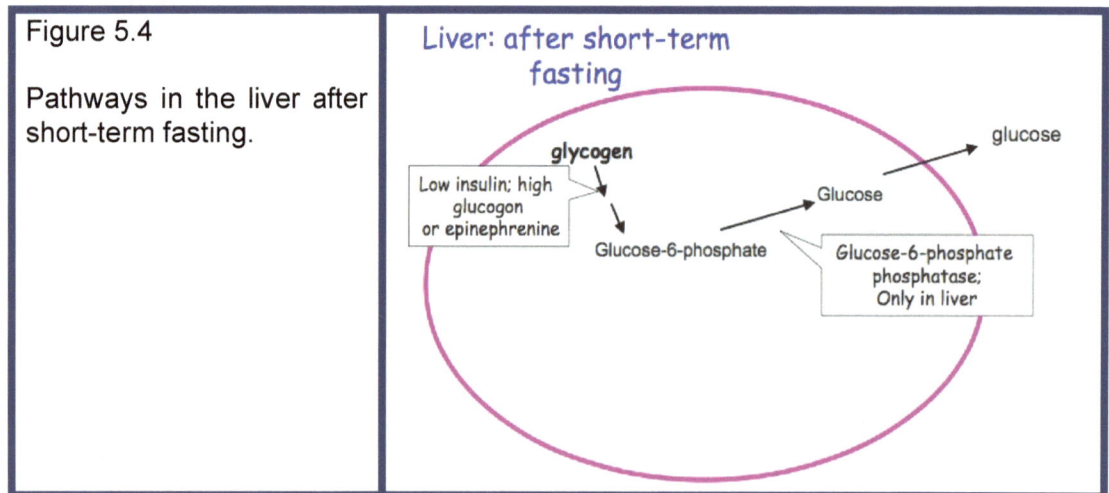

Figure 5.4

Pathways in the liver after short-term fasting.

An enzyme called "glucose-6-phosphate phosphatase" (a long name!) catalyzes the final step in getting glucose from glucose-6-phosphate. "Phosphatase" refers to an enzyme that breaks off phosphate, and the name of the enzyme means that it breaks off phosphate from glucose-6-phosphate.[6]

This enzyme is found in the liver. Other tissues do not have this enzyme, and so once glucose has a phosphate on it, in other tissues this glucose stays within the cells. (There is an exception: a small amount of this enzyme is in the kidney, and the kidney supplies some glucose in long term fasting. We will discuss this in the next chapter). Consequently, other tissues use glycogen as an energy store only for themselves. Since they do have the enzyme glucose-6-phosphate phosphatase they cannot release glucose into the blood stream for the use of other tissues.

So this is why we call the liver "the good guy". It releases glucose from its glycogen stores into the blood for the brain to use.

The enzymes that release glucose from glycogen are also triggered to act in an emergency by the hormone epinephrine. We mentioned before that GB is walking in the woods and a bear jumps out. The hormone epinephrine (aka adrenaline) comes into play. Epinephrine stimulates the break-down of glycogen in both the liver and muscle. The glycogen from the muscle gets metabolized to lactate in the anaerobic, fast muscles. Glucose goes to CO_2 in the aerobic muscles. Both muscle types will be used when GB runs away. GB is saved!

5.5.2 Why and when muscle uses its stored glycogen

Muscles attached to our skeleton enable us to move, search for food, escape danger and do work. Muscles consume much of our bodies' energy. A person who is rigorously skiing, running or swimming consumes up to 6000 kcal/day. When this person is sedentary, the amount of calories consumed is about 1500 kcal/day or even less. From this it is clear that muscles consume a lot of ATP when we are active – and they must be ready for sudden action at all times.

Muscles are biological engineering marvels. Muscle cells have many fibers and the fibers are composed mainly of two proteins, called actin and myosin; both of these form filaments. When muscles are relaxed, the filament composed of actin molecules and the filament composed of myosin molecules do not interact with each other. When muscle contracts, a portion of the myosin binds to actin. To bind, energy is required, and ATP is used. As the muscle contracts, the portion of myosin "walks" along the actin, much like a caterpillar walking. This makes the muscle shorter, and the muscle pulls upon a bone causing it to move.

---

[6] Remember that the names of many enzymes end in "-ase".

Figure 5.5. How muscles work. When muscle is relaxed, actin and myosin filaments are non-interacting. When muscle contracts, actin and myosin interact. The molecules of myosin bind to actin. For this to occur, ATP must be used.	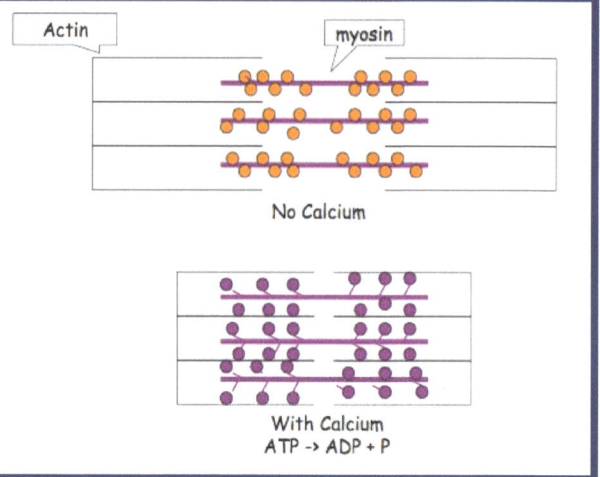

What makes muscle contract? Muscle contracts in response to nerve stimulation. Nerves cause the release of calcium (Ca) from specialized organelles in the muscle cell. (These membranes are the endoplasmic reticulum organelles, see Figure 1 in Chapter 3). In response to the presence of Ca, ATP is hydrolyzed by myosin, to form ADP and P, and the muscle contracts. When the muscle is no longer stimulated, Ca gets pumped back into the membranous organelle, and the muscle relaxes. It is again extended.

The function of the amazing muscles is related to metabolism. There are two basic types of skeletal muscles: fast and slow. Without resorting to autopsy of humans, we can illustrate these two muscle types during our Thanksgiving dinner. The wild turkey, which is the progenitor of our domestic turkey, has a mixture of red and white muscle on its breast. In the domestic turkey, there is a selection for white muscle, so that we can have white meat for dinner. White muscles are called "fast muscle". The wild turkey survives by flying rapidly to cover when a predator is near-by. It accomplishes this using the fast muscle on its breast for flight. The white muscles use glycolysis to make ATP. On the other hand, when the turkey is picking up corn from the ground, it needs to stand for a long time. It uses the "slow muscles". The leg of turkey has predominantly red muscles, they contain many mitochondria, and a red protein, called myoglobin that makes the muscle red and serves to transport O_2 in the cells. Fat is the main fuel of red muscles and oxidative phosphorylation is used to make ATP in the slow muscles.

Fast muscles use glycolysis for energy; and they work in quick response to stimuli. Fast muscles are full of glycogen. Under stimulation, glycogen breaks down to glucose, which gets transformed into lactate with the formation of ATP via the glycolysis pathway.

Now comes the neat thing. Nerve stimulation causes the release of Ca from the endoplasmic reticulum, and the Ca causes myosin and actin to interact and the muscle contracts. This very same Ca stimulates the break-down of glycogen to form glucose-6-phosphate. If you are texting while you are reading this, the white muscle fibers in your figures are being stimulated to contract by Ca, which also stimulates a little squirt of glucose-6-phosphate to come from glycogen, and then this glucose is used to produce ATP in the fiber. As we noted above, epinephrine also stimulates the breakdown of glycogen in muscle. This also quickly produces glucose-6-phosphate in the white muscle cells, for a quick response for movement.

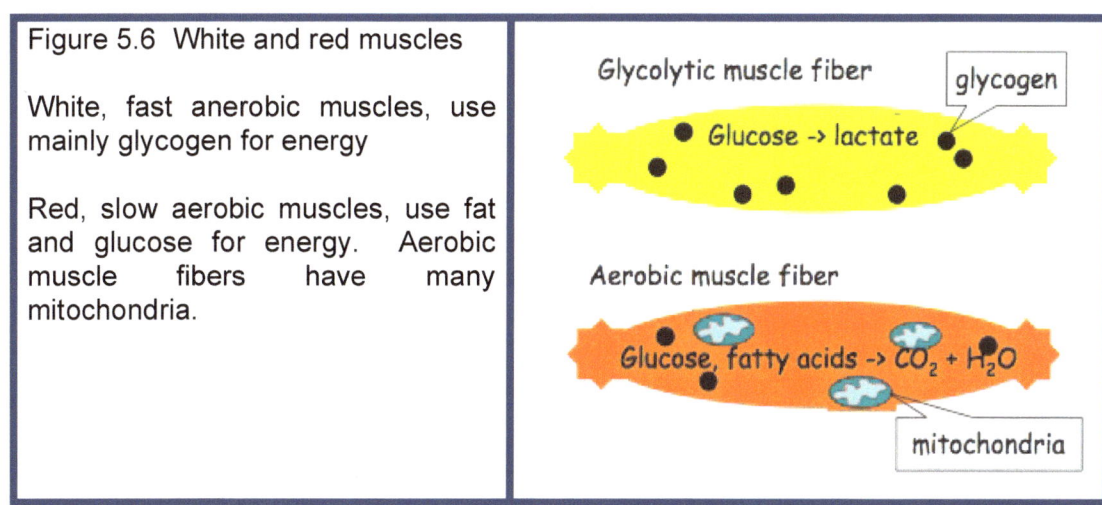

Figure 5.6 White and red muscles

White, fast anaerobic muscles, use mainly glycogen for energy

Red, slow aerobic muscles, use fat and glucose for energy. Aerobic muscle fibers have many mitochondria.

Glycolytic muscle fiber
glycogen
Glucose -> lactate

Aerobic muscle fiber
Glucose, fatty acids -> CO_2 + H_2O
mitochondria

Figure 5.7 gives summary of the metabolism in muscle during exercise. After anerobic exercise lactate that builds up in the muscle, gradually leaks out.

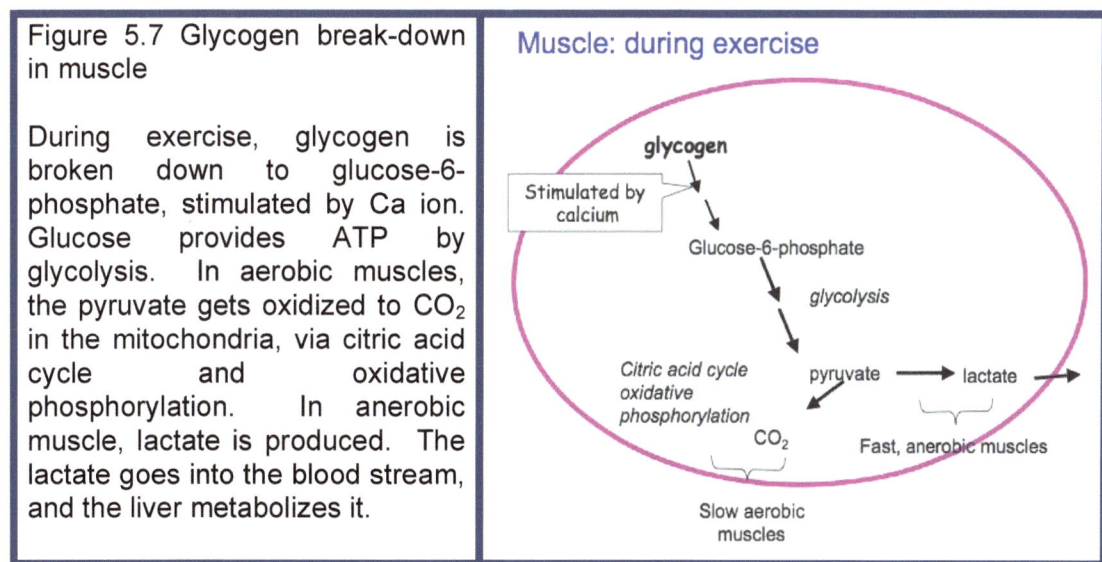

Figure 5.7 Glycogen break-down in muscle

During exercise, glycogen is broken down to glucose-6-phosphate, stimulated by Ca ion. Glucose provides ATP by glycolysis. In aerobic muscles, the pyruvate gets oxidized to CO_2 in the mitochondria, via citric acid cycle and oxidative phosphorylation. In anaerobic muscle, lactate is produced. The lactate goes into the blood stream, and the liver metabolizes it.

Muscle: during exercise
glycogen
Stimulated by calcium
Glucose-6-phosphate
glycolysis
Citric acid cycle oxidative phosphorylation
pyruvate ⟶ lactate
CO_2
Fast, anaerobic muscles
Slow aerobic muscles

In humans, the aerobic and the glycolytic fibers are mixed together in each muscle type. Sprinters and weight lifters tend to have high content of glycolytic muscle fibers, which allow them to exert a burst of work for a short period of time. People who specialize in sports that require long sustained effort have muscles with high content of aerobic muscles that use fat as the primary fuel source. Humans can outrun most animals and if we train, we are able to run long distances for long periods of time. Tarahumara people from Mexico can run over 400 miles up and down canyons in a period of two days. We would expect that their muscles would be rich in mitochondria, and that during running the major source of energy would be coming from fat, not the glycogen stores.

5.6. Summary: Hormones regulate the storage and retrieval of glycogen

Two major concepts are introduced in this chapter. The first concept in this chapter is that hormones regulate storage and retrieval of food molecules. The second major concept explains why hormone regulation is so important. The important concept is that the storage and release of a fuel depends upon the organ. We saw that glycogen is used differently in liver and in muscle.

High level of insulin stimulates the enzymes that contribute to the storage of glucose in the form of glycogen. Low levels of insulin and high level of glucogon stimulates the enzymes that catalyze glycogen breakdown back to glucose. The breakdown is further stimulated by adrenaline in both liver and muscle and by Ca^{++} in muscle.

In this book we are emphasizing basic concepts. A theme is that there are key enzymes that when either stimulated or inhibited control which pathway is working. In case of glycogen, the substances that stimulate synthesis, inhibit break-down, and vice versa. If you take an advanced course in Biochemistry, you will be given greater detail about how hormones affect particular enzymes. To whet your appetite for further study, at the end of the chapter is a summary of the hormonal regulation by insulin of glycogen synthesis and glycolysis.

5.7. Clinical case

This case illustrates what happens when glucose cannot be stored as glycogen, or retrieved from storage.

Case: muscle wasting in the hand (Based on: Brunberg et al. Arch. Neurol. 25, 171-178, 1971 and Murase et al. J. Neurol. Sciences 20 287-295, 1973.)

ST is a 43 year-old male patient, who in the past few years has had episodes of aching fingers, stiffness of legs and arms and suffers from general weakness. He noticed that the muscles in his hand show atrophy – i.e., they are wasting away. Indeed, the physician estimated about a 30 – 60% decrease in overall muscle strength.

His blood chemistry showed some deviations from normal. After an 8 hour fast the blood glucose was 3 to 3.5 mM (normal control: 4 to 4.5 mM). In the hospital after another 8 hour fast, keto-acids were detected in the urine. (Keto-acids are made from fatty acids and they are normally made under long-term starvation conditions. The presence of keto-acids indicates that fat is being used as fuel. This will be described in Chapter 7).

In order to study why ST had a low amount of glucose in blood after not eating for 8 hours, the physicians ordered a glucose tolerance test. In a glucose tolerance test, the patient first fasts overnight, and then drinks a drink containing 100 grams of glucose. Following the drink, samples of his blood are taken and analyzed for glucose. Here is the result of the glucose tolerance test.

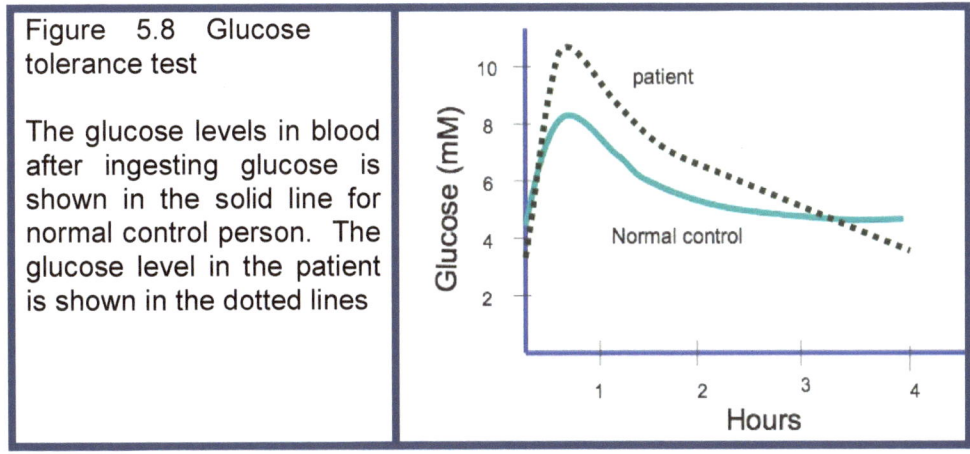

Figure 5.8 Glucose tolerance test The glucose levels in blood after ingesting glucose is shown in the solid line for normal control person. The glucose level in the patient is shown in the dotted lines

Diagnosis and Comments: This patient, ST, was found to be deficient in an enzyme required for the breakdown of glycogen. The enzyme that was deficient is the same in liver and muscle. So both the liver and muscles are affected.

So we now ask how the impaired enzyme is affecting ST. The weakness and wasting of muscle is consistent with low ATP. In this patient, ATP is low during anaerobic exercise. He cannot release glucose from glycogen, and therefore glycolysis is impaired, because glucose-6-phosphate is not being made from glycogen. The patient noticed wasting of muscles in his hands. The muscles in the hands are rich in white muscle fiber, and these muscles rely on glycolysis to make ATP.

In a normal person after eating an excess of glucose, glucose concentration in the blood increases. Insulin is released and insulin stimulates the removal of glucose. As glucose levels drops, the level of the hormone glucogon increases. Glucogon stimulates the breakdown of glycogen from the liver. The glucose released from liver glycogon goes into the blood, and blood glucose levels remain constant.

In ST, giving glucose causes an increase in glucose levels in the blood that is larger than seen in the controls. The reason for this, glucose is not being made into glycogen because the glycogen levels are already full (because the enzyme to breakdown glycogen is missing). At long times after taking glucose, the level of glucose in ST's blood is below that seen in the control patient. That is because glycogen in the liver cannot be broken down to glucose.

A question for you to think about: what would you do for this patient?

5.8 For further study

Figure 5.8 enzymes that are the major points of regulation for glycolysis and glycogen synthesis.

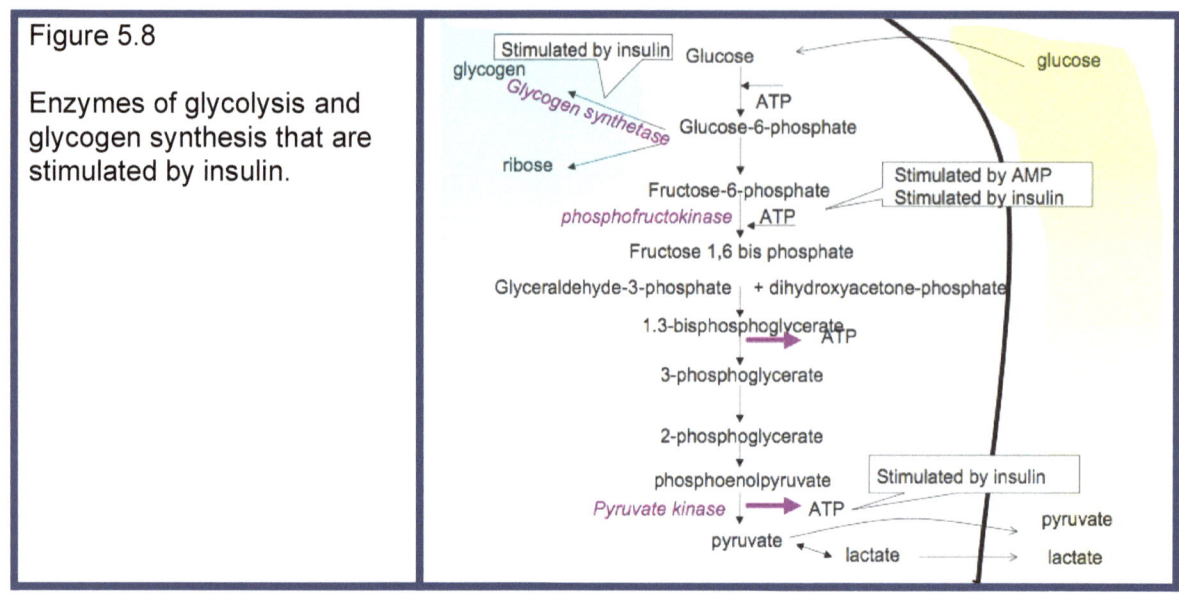

Figure 5.8

Enzymes of glycolysis and glycogen synthesis that are stimulated by insulin.

Glycogen synthetase: It is indirectly stimulated by insulin. Insulin inhibits the formation of cyclic AMP. At low cyclic AMP, synthetase is active. (High cyclic AMP, the enzyme that breaks down glycogen is activated).

Phosphofructokinase: AMP stimulates this enzyme; AMP is high when ATP is low, so AMP serves to "tell" this enzyme that more ATP is needed. Phophosfructokinase is also stimulated by 2,6 frutobisphosphate, a compound that is high at when insulin levels are high and glucogon levels are low (I/G is high).

Pyruvate kinase: Pyruvate kinase is inhibited by having a phosphate put on the enzyme. At high I/G proteins called protein phosphorylases are stimulated. These proteins remove phosphate from pyruvate kinase, and pyruvate kinase is stimulated.

6. Sugar is made from proteins and small molecules; toxic N is removed

6.1 Our bodies keep blood sugar levels from dropping during fasting by making glucose from other molecules

In the past chapter, we saw how liver glycogen maintained glucose levels. But, even after glycogen is depleted, blood glucose does not drop to zero. If we were to follow the concentration of sugar in GBs blood, we would find that his blood sugar only gradually declines, even when most of liver glycogen is gone.

Figure 6.1
Sugar levels in the blood after eating and during fasting. After eating glucose in blood rises due to influx of glucose from the diet. This glucose is taken into cells. After this spike, glucose levels only slowly declines. Initially glucose is released from liver glycogen and then from liver using gluconeogenesis. In gluconeogenesis, liver makes glucose from amino acids.

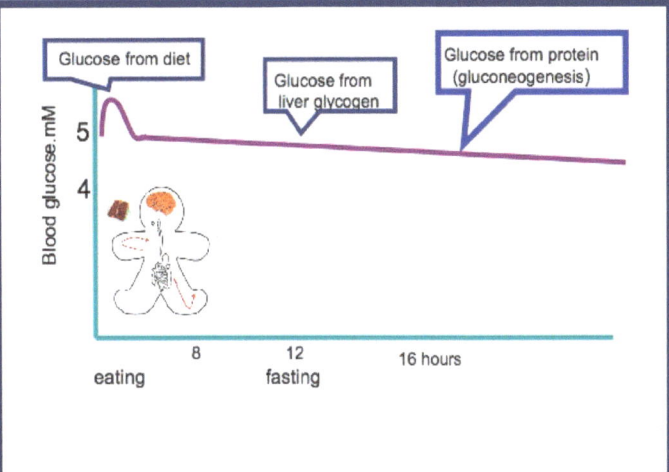

When glycogen is gone, where does glucose come from? It turns out that liver and, to a lesser amount kidney, makes glucose from amino acids of proteins and other small molecules. Making glucose is called **gluconeogenesis** (genesis means "to make" and "neo" means new, so this word means making new glucose). Gluconeogenesis in GB occurs when glucose from diet and glucose from glycogen is depleted, as in an overnight and longer fasting.

Table 6.1 lists most of the small molecules that can be made into glucose. One part of this chapter is about how these small molecules make glucose, to give "fuel", in the form of glucose to the brain.

Table 6.1. Molecules that are used to make glucose

Gluconeogenic compounds	Structure	Source and use
alanine		From protein. Liver uses mainly alanine for gluconeogenesis
Glutamate/glutamine		From protein. Liver and kidney use for glutamate and glutamine for gluconeogenesis
Pyruvate/ lactate		Lactate is formed from glycogen by anaerobic muscle during exercise. Lactate and pyruvate is also formed from glucose via glycolysis in red blood cells (RBC's).
glycerol		Part of fat, i.e. triglyceride. Glycerol is a significant source of C for gluconeogensis during long term starvation

As for metabolism of all food, regulation of gluconeogenesis is achieved by hormones. In the previous chapter we introduced epinephrine and glucogon, two hormones that play a role in the release of glucose from glycogen. In this chapter some functions of the hormone **cortisol** are introduced. Among its functions, cortisol regulates the breakdown of protein and its conversion into glucose. So along with epinephrine and glucogon, cortisol is counter-regulatory to insulin. Insulin acts to reduce glucose in the blood. Cortisol, epinephrine and glucogon act together to restore glucose levels in the blood.

Table 2 gives a tally of these hormones, and the influence blood glucose levels on their secretion.

Table 2. Hormones during high and low glucose

Blood glucose, mmol/l	Hormone response	Metabolic pathways
> 8	Exceeds renal threshold, and glucose is lost in the urine, along with water, and electrolytes (Na^+ and K^+). Insulin high	
5.5	**Insulin** secretion increases as sugar levels increase	Glycolysis, glycogen synthesis, fat synthesis, protein synthesis
4.6	Insulin secretion decreases, but does not go to zero	
3.8	Increased secretion of **glucagon** and **epinephrine**	Glucagon stimulates glycogen breakdown in liver; Epinephrine stimulates glycogen breakdown in liver and muscle
3.2	**Cortisol** secretion	Muscle protein break-down; gluconeogenesis

The other part of this chapter is how to deal with a by-product of protein metabolism. Our proteins are always being broken down and remade. Proteins are made from amino acids and they are composed of C, H, O and N. The N released when our proteins are broken down produces ammonia (NH_3). Excess protein from diet also makes NH_3 and bacteria in the intestine make NH_3. Ammonia is very toxic. Therefore, in the discussion on protein metabolism, we must also talk about how N is removed in the body.

There are two ways the body gets rid of ammonia. The most important way is that it is transformed into urea (NH_3CONH_3) in the liver. Urea produced by the liver goes into the blood stream, and the kidney excretes it into the urine. Under long-term starvation, there is another way to get rid of excess N. The kidney produces ammonia from glutamate and glutamine, and ammonia is excreted into the urine. During this time, the C's of glutamate and glutamine are converted into glucose by the kidney.

6.2 Overview of glucose production in liver and kidney during fasting

This part of the book may be the most shocking – we make glucose from protein! So before we compare metabolism in liver and kidney, let us get an overview of when and how much glucose the two organs produce. As glycogen gets depleted in the liver, liver steps up its production of new glucose. The production of glucose, in kidney, in contrast is increased during long-term fasting, i.e. starvation. The time-course and source of C's for glucose production are shown in Figures 6.2 and 6.3.

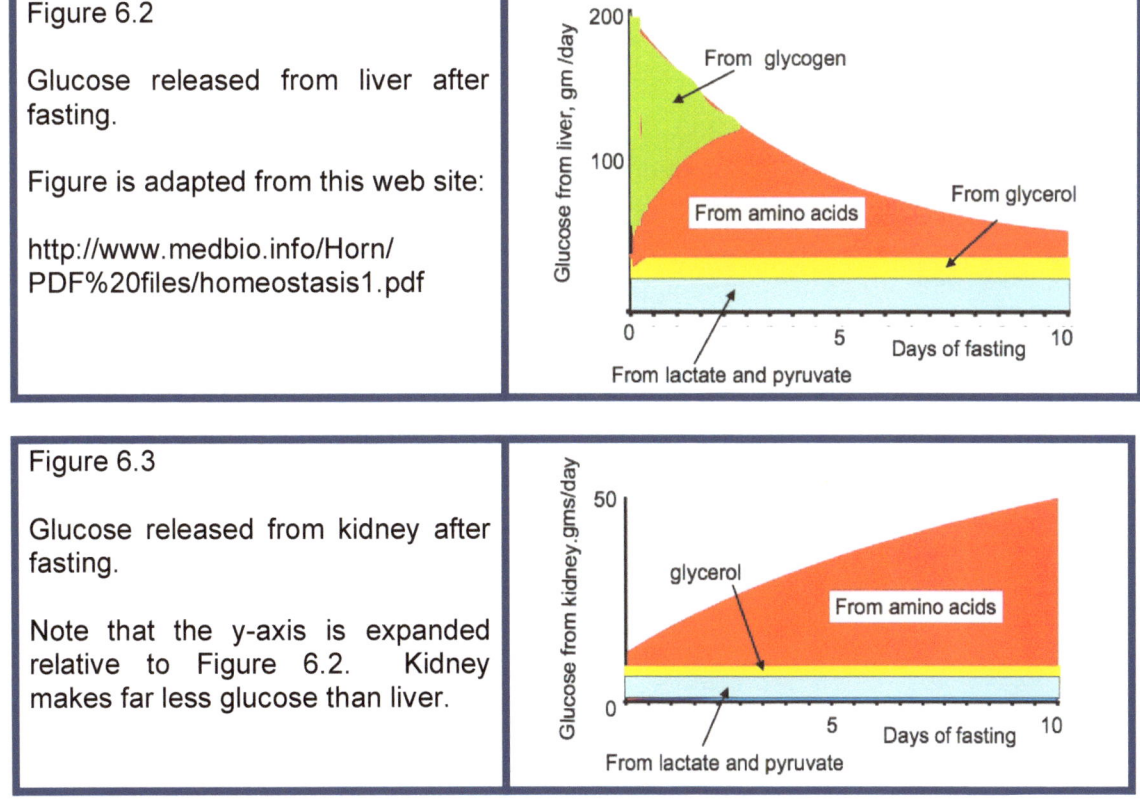

Figure 6.2

Glucose released from liver after fasting.

Figure is adapted from this web site:

http://www.medbio.info/Horn/PDF%20files/homeostasis1.pdf

Figure 6.3

Glucose released from kidney after fasting.

Note that the y-axis is expanded relative to Figure 6.2.   Kidney makes far less glucose than liver.

Here are some things to notice about these graphs:

1. When glucose from glycogen goes down, liver steps up the production of glucose from amino acids. It turns out that the amino acid alanine is the major source of C's to make glucose.

2. The production of glucose from amino acids in the liver declines after several days of fasting. In the next chapter we will learn why. (Hint: In long-term fasting, ketoacids are made from fatty acids, and the brain uses this as fuel. Glucose is no longer the major fuel for brain and the break-down of protein is reduced.)

3. The kidney steps up production of glucose after long-term fasting. The different time course of making glucose tells us that the liver and kidney make glucose for different reasons. As will be explained below, the major sources of C's for making glucose by the kidney are glutamine and glutamate. These amino acids release NH_3, and this serves to adjust the pH of urine during starvation.

4. Glycerol serves to make glucose in both liver and kidney. Glycerol comes from triglyceride, fat.

5. Lactate and pyruvate are made into glucose in both organs. These substances are produced by glycolysis in red blood cells (RBC's). Since all lactate and pyruvate is made back into glucose, RBC's in effect do not use up glucose nor contribute to net glucose levels in blood.

Figure 6.2 does not show what is happening during exercise by anaerobic muscle. In anaerobic exercise, glycogen is broken down to glucose-1-phosphate, which gets converted to lactate, via glycolysis. Lactate goes into the blood, and the liver uses this lactate to make glucose.

6. Under short-term fasting conditions, the amount of glucose produced by the kidney is less than 20% of the total, but during long-term starvation, the kidney production of glucose can equal that of the liver.

6.3 Sugar from glycerol

We will describe the use of glycerol and pyruvate/lactate to make glucose first, and then discuss the more significant use of protein as a precursor for making glucose.

A small amount of the C's in sugar made by gluconeogenesis is obtained from fat. This is a fat molecule, also known as triglyceride:

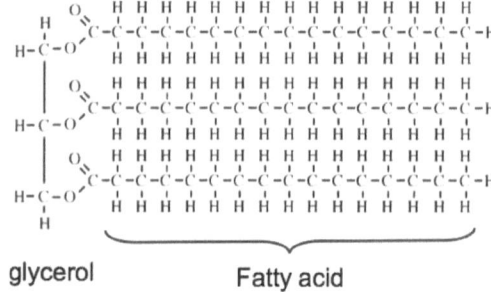

glycerol   Fatty acid

When fat is broken down, it splits into fatty acids and glycerol. Fatty acids go to 2 C units and are not made into glucose. But glycerol, which is 3 C is also part of fat. When fat is being made, glycerol, a side product of glycolysis, is used. This glycerol part is used when fat is being broken down to made glucose.

Figure 6.4	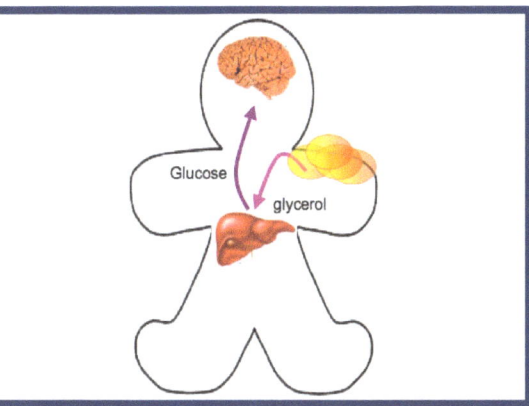
Fat is broken down into fatty acids and glycerol. Glycerol is made into glucose in the liver, and from there glucose goes into the blood stream.	

Figure 6.5 shows the pathway for making glucose from glycerol. In the cytoplasm the 3 C molecule combines with another 3 C molecule to produce 6 C molecule, glucose 6-phosphate. The final step is that glucose-6-phosphate loses its phosphate and glucose is formed. This enzyme is only found in the liver and kidney, and so these are only organs that make glucose.

Figure 6.5	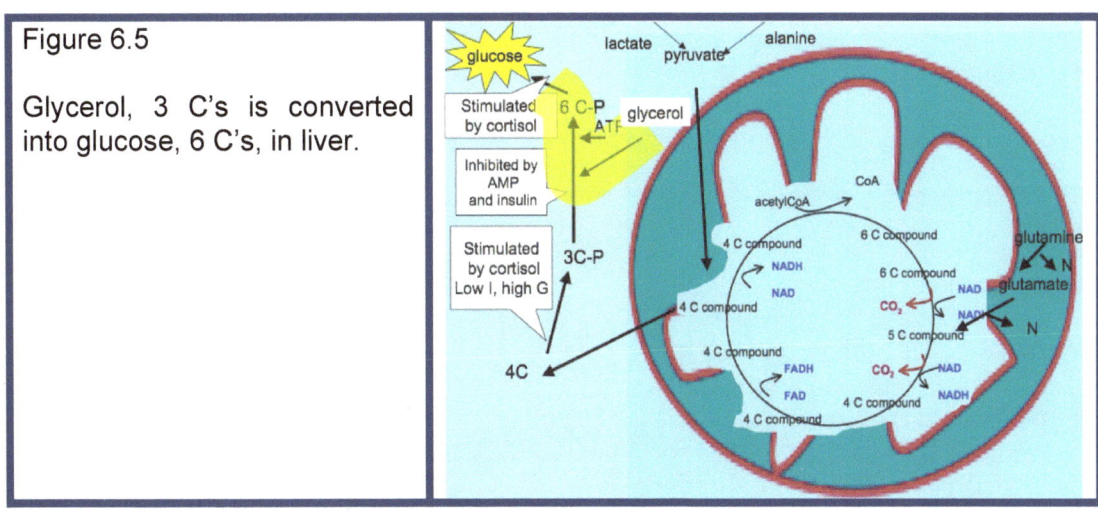
Glycerol, 3 C's is converted into glucose, 6 C's, in liver.	

Since fat is always being used, the amount of glycerol made into glucose is relatively constant over the period of starvation (Figures 6.2 and 6.3). But during many days of fasting, the overall production of glucose from the liver decreases (Figure 6.2). Then the percentage of glucose obtained from glycerol becomes more significant.

6.4 Sugar from lactate and pyruvate

Lactate and pyruvate (both 3 C's) are made from glucose. Lactate is formed from glycogen in anaerobic muscles during strenuous exercise. Lactate and pyruvate are always being made from glucose in RBC's by glycolysis since glycolysis provides ATP for RBC's. Without ATP the cells would break.

Lactate from muscle and RBC's goes into the blood circulation, and is taken in by the liver, which can make it into glucose. This glucose goes into the blood circulation and can be used by other tissues, including the brain, or can be recycled back to the tissues that originally produced lactate.

Figure 6.6	
Glucose is used in RBC's to make ATP by glycolysis. The products are 3 C compounds, pyruvate and lactate. The liver makes glucose from pyruvate and lactate, but the amount of glucose made is equal to the amount broken down in RBC. So this process recycles glucose but makes no extra.	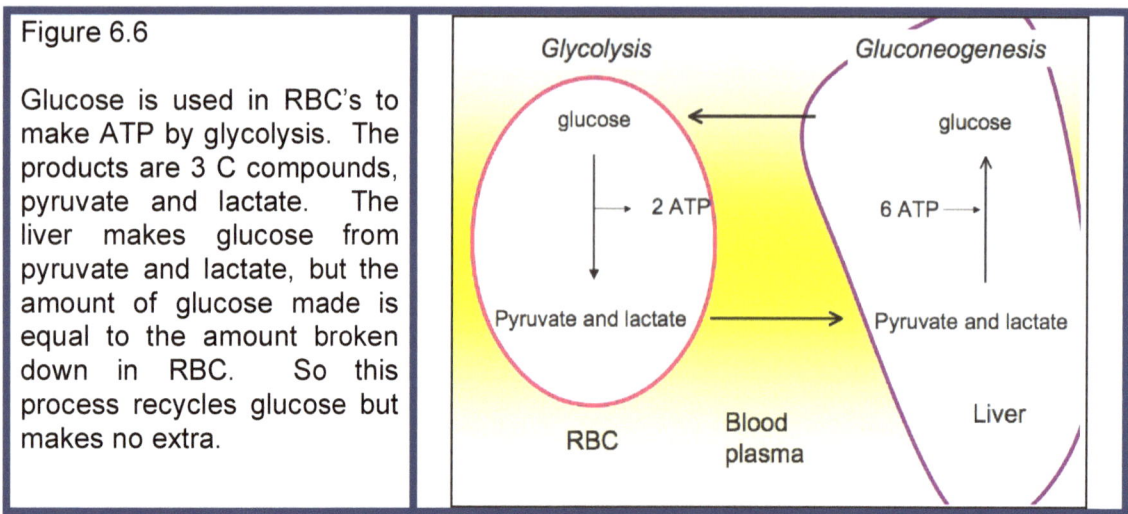

For RBC's, there is no net glucose gained or lost by this process, so RBC's do not supply lactate to make glucose for the brain. In muscle, the possible amount of lactate available to make glucose is limited by the amount of glycogen.

Here is the pathway for making glucose from lactate and pyruvate:

Figure 6.7	
Lactate is made into glucose in the liver. First, lactate is converted to pyruvate. A C is added to make a 4 C compound. This compound exits the mitochondrion, and the C is removed and a phosphate is added. The 3 C compound adds to another 3 C compound and glucose-6-phosphate is eventually made. The phosphate is removed to make glucose.	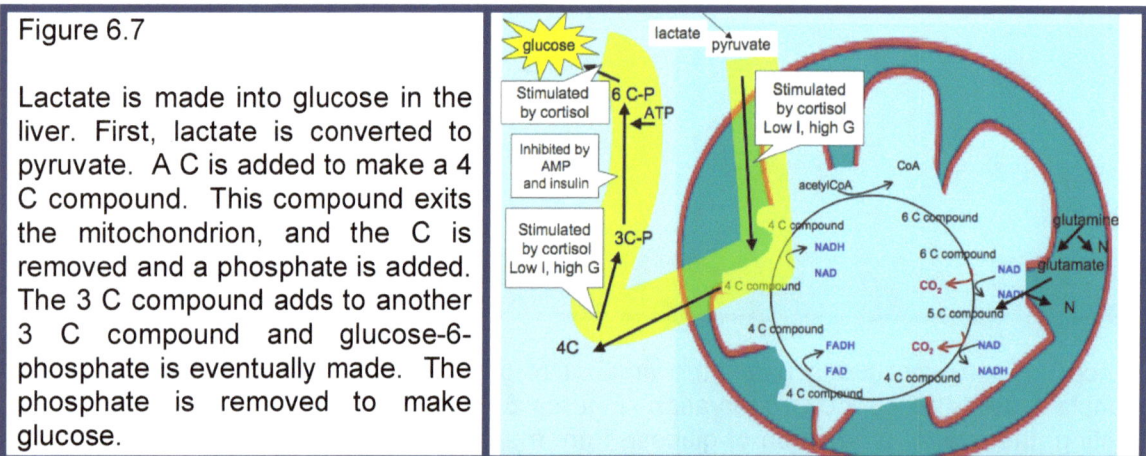

6.5 Roles of proteins in the body

Now we are getting to that important idea that proteins can be made into glucose. "Everyone" knows that fat accumulates when we eat too much, and fat is diminished when we eat less. Athletes know the importance of glycogen in athletic efforts. Marathon runners attempt to increase their glycogen stores by eating carbohydrates the night before a race. But, how many people realize that protein is converted into sugar, and that this conversion occurs normally during every day?

Unlike glycogen and fat, which are storage forms of food, there is no storage form of protein that just sits there and does nothing except wait to be metabolized. All protein in our bodies has uses. Yet, proteins play an important role in nutrition and are used to supply energy. Proteins that we eat, whether the protein comes from plants or animals, are broken down to amino acids in the intestine, and these amino acids are used to make the proteins of our body. When excess protein is eaten, the amino acids are transformed into fat and glucose in the form of glycogen. During fasting, protein of our body is used as fuel for energy. We have emphasized the importance of glucose in brain metabolism. During fasting, the same proteins that enable us to move, transport ions and many other things are converted into glucose by the liver. The kidney also makes glucose from amino acids, but the regulation of gluconeogenesis is different in liver and kidney.

6.6 Amino acids are involved in gluconeogenesis

Because new proteins are always being made we absolutely need to eat proteins in order to survive. Proteins contain 20 different amino acids. The sequence of amino acids determines the function of the protein. The proteins within all cells that have mitochondria are made within the cell from amino acids from the blood.

The metabolism of each amino acid is unique, but nearly all amino acids can be made into sugar. All organs and cells contain proteins. Muscle tissue has the largest amount of proteins in the body. Muscle proteins are always being made and being degraded. A typical lifetime for a muscle protein is about 10 days. That means that about 7% of muscle proteins are broken down and remade in a day. During fasting more protein is broken down than is remade. Although all amino acids are released when protein is broken down, enzymes in muscle convert them so that the major amino acids released into the blood are alanine, glutamate and glutamine.

Alanine has 3 C's and it is a derivative of propionate and is related to pyruvate:

Alanine is termed a "non-essential" amino acid. This means that it can be made in the body from other components. For instance, alanine can be made from pyruvate, using the N from another amino acid. This reaction can also be reversed: alanine can be made into pyruvate by giving the amino group to another molecule. This is the reaction:

| Amino acid | pyruvate | | alanine |

In this equation R stands for any amino acid. This equation says that another amino acid can give its amino group to pyruvate; in so doing alanine is formed. The double arrow also indicates that alanine can be used to form amino acids too. The amino group of alanine can be put on the "R"- acid, to get an amino acid and pyruvate. Since all 20 amino acids are needed to make proteins, and each protein molecule is made of a definite sequence of amino acids, this swapping of amino groups helps to have the right ratio of amino acids available for making proteins.

Glutamate is another amino acid that is made in the body and hence it is also classified as a non-essential amino acid. Glutamate has five C's and two carboxyl groups.

In the citric acid cycle (Chapter 5), we indicated some compounds with 5 C's. When glutamate loses its amino group it becomes one of these 5 C compounds. You may be familiar with glutamate as a food additive – monosodium glutamate. Glutamate is a common amino acid, found in most proteins.

The final non-essential amino acid that we discuss is glutamine. This is glutamine:

Glutamine is like glutamate except that it has an amino group where glutamate has OH. Notice that glutamine has two N's. This is important because glutamine helps to get rid of excess N.

Alanine, glutamate and glutamine are used to transport N from the various tissues to the liver, where the excretion product of N, urea, is made. Their carbons can be made into glucose. Glutamine also brings N to the kidney, where NH_3 is formed.

6.7 Amino acids made into sugar

We have seen the fate of fatty acid metabolism: formation of the 2 C unit, acetylCoA, which gets metabolized in the mitochondria to CO_2 to form ATP. Fatty acids are not converted into glucose. 2 C units are not converted into 3C units, and 3 C units are required to make glucose, which is a 6 C compound.

Figure 6.8 shows the sources for C for glucose when GB does not eat.

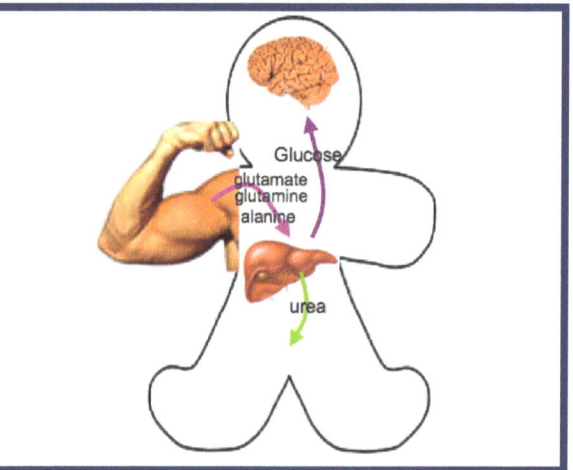

Figure 6.8

Protein, mainly from muscle, is broken down into amino acids. The major amino acids that are released are alanine, glutamate and glutamine. Liver and, to a lesser extent, kidney make these amino acids into glucose. The extra N atoms are made into urea by the liver. The urea is excreted in the urine,

The amino acids are converted into glucose by the scheme in Figure 6.9. Alanine gets converted into pyruvate. During eating conditions, the enzyme that breaks alanine into two C's is activated. During fasting, cortisol is high, glucogon is high and insulin is low. These conditions stimulate an enzyme that puts 1 C on pyruvate to make a 4 C compound. This compound exits the mitochondria. The enzyme that converts the 4 C into 3 C is stimulated by cortisol, as is the other enzymes that make glucose.

Figure 6.9 Making glucose from alanine, pyruvate .

The figure also indicates that cortisol stimulates the enzymes of gluconeogenesis in the liver.

Note that this figure is identical to Figure 6.7, except for the addition of allanine at the top.

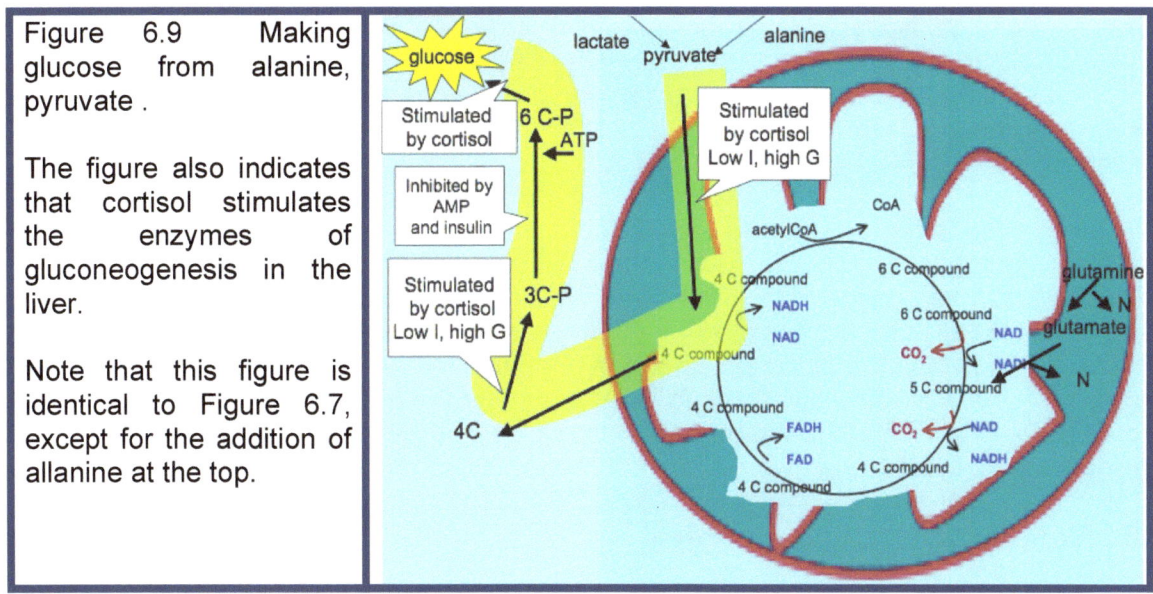

Glutamate and glutamine are the other amino acids involved in gluconeogenesis. The metabolism of glutamate and glutamine uses some of the reactions of the citric acid cycle (Chapter 4). The pathway is shown in the figure below.

Figure 6.10

Glutamine and glutamate, products of protein breakdown in muscle, ultimately gets made into glucose in the liver. This same pathway is used by the kidney.

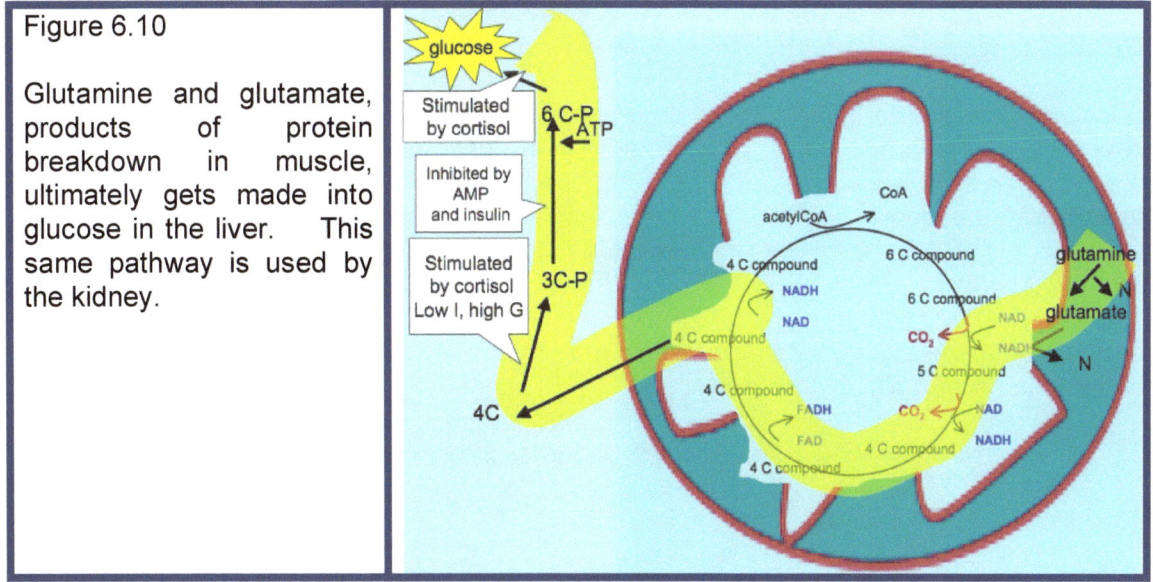

Glutamine, which is C 5, first loses one N group to form glutamate, and then it loses the other N to form a 5 C compound in the mitochondria. This compound loses CO_2, and forms NADH and FADH in a series of chemical reactions. Remember that NADH and FADH are used in oxidative phosphorylation to make ATP. The 4 C compounds undergo reaction and one of them comes out of the mitochondria. In the cytoplasm, the 4 C compound loses CO_2, and becomes 3C. From then on, gluconeogenesis in the cytoplasm takes over.

6.8 Hormones regulate the production of glucose from amino acids

The hormone cortisol stimulates the making of enzymes that catalyzes reactions in the cytoplasm that changes 4C to 3C. In this way, cortisol stimulates the breakdown of some proteins to produce the starting materials for gluconeogenesis (alanine, glutamine and glutamate) and the synthesis of other proteins that aid in making these amino acids into glucose.

When glucose is broken down to the 3 C compounds pyruvate and lactate in glycolysis, ATP is formed. When 3 C compound is used to make glucose, energy, ATP, is required. This ATP can be coming from the metabolism of amino acids themselves. We noticed above that the metabolism of glutamine produces NADH and FADH, which can be used to make ATP. But during gluconeogenesis ATP mainly comes from the oxidation of fatty acids. They are broken down to acetylCoA, and enter the mitochondria, and are oxidized to CO_2, forming ATP. So, although fatty acids do not give C's to make glucose, their oxidation provides the energy for glucose formation by giving ATP.

6.9 What to do with waste N: Liver

At all times, in sickness or health and under feeding or starvation, proteins are being made and degraded. Some proteins last for a long time – up to our lifetime; the protein molecules in the lens of the eye are as old as our age. Some proteins survive a short time, only hours or even minutes. For example, PEP carboxykinase, the main enzyme that regulates making glucose, is synthesized when cortisol is high, but it is constantly being degraded. When feeding occurs, the levels of PEP carboxykinase drop rapidly, because cortisol levels fall and the enzyme is no longer being made.

Because proteins are being broken down continually, at all times we need to be making new protein. The amino acids from one protein are used to make another proteins. Since the amino acids generated when a certain protein is degraded may not exactly contain the amino acids needed to synthesize a different protein, at all times in our lives we need to eat some protein. The N's from the excess amino acids need to be removed.

The liver is once again the "good guy" in that it removes N's. Ammonia (NH_3) is generated from glutamine and glutamate and then this ammonia reacts with CO_2 and ATP to form a compound called carbamyl-phosphate.

$$NH_3 + CO_2 + 2\ ATP \rightarrow carbamyl\ phosphate + 2\ ADP$$

This is carbamyl phosphate:

Carbamyl phosphate has one N and 1 C.

Carbamyl phosphate picks up a nitrogen atom from another amino acid in a series of reactions, called the urea cycle. Most of these reactions occur in the mitochondria.

Finally urea is formed. This is urea:

$$H_2N-\overset{\overset{\displaystyle O}{\|}}{C}-NH_2$$

Urea goes into the blood. Kidneys take the urea from the blood, and the urea is excreted in urine.

The urea cycle.is operating at all times, because protein degradation and synthesis is occurring at all times. If your diet is high in protein, more N is removed by the urea cycle, because the excess N from the amino acids must be disposed of.

6.10 N is released when glutamate and glutamine are metabolized in kidney

Figure 6.11

Kidney uses glutamine and glutamate to produce glucose during long-term starvation.

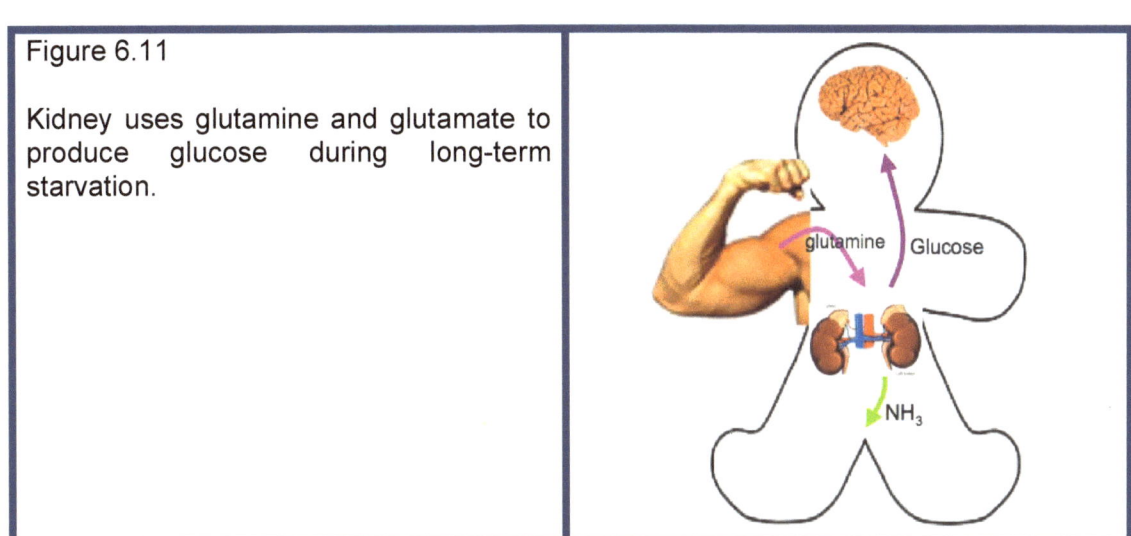

During prolonged starvation fat is gradually used up, and then there is severe protein breakdown. Eventually, liver cannot make all extra N into urea. This is when gluconeogenesis in the kidney becomes important.

The kidney takes in glutamine and converts it to glutamate, releasing NH_3. This is the reaction:

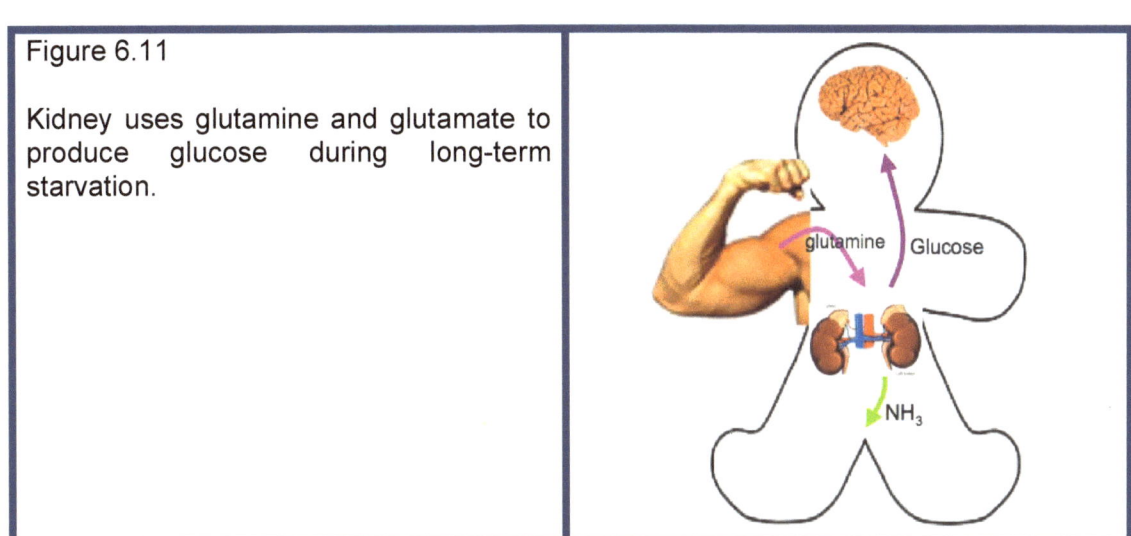

Then the amino group of glutamate is also removed to yield NH_3 and a 5 C compound. This compound is made into glucose as in Figure 6.11. NH_3 is released into the urine. We will see that during long starvation, acids are formed, and some of these leak into the urine. NH_3 helps to keep the pH of the urine to the proper value.

6.11 Protein breakdown in disease

Protein breakdown occurs during many diseases. Viral infection stimulates protein breakdown from muscle. You may have felt weak after flu (caused by a virus), even after the infection is gone. A patient with HIV (also a virus disease) often suffers from wasting of muscle. Presumably, protein breakdown serves to give amino acids, which are used to form antibodies that fight the infection. Also, mucus – the scourge of sinus infections – is largely made of carbohydrate. If you are not eating during a cold, this carbohydrate is made from protein.

There are brain-body interactions regarding protein metabolism too. Cortisol is higher in stress. Long-term high level of cortisol leads to general loss of strength, as muscle is broken down. Many people complain that they tend to get colds or other infections during stressful times. Long-term high levels of cortisol can ultimately reduce the levels of antibodies, proteins made in white blood cells that help ward off infection.

6.12 Hormonal regulation of protein breakdown and gluconeogenesis

Life is not simple. The production of cortisol is regulated by a series of other hormones. When glycogen stores in the muscle are close to depletion, the hypothalamus in the brain secretes a hormone called CRF (Corticotropin-Releasing Factor). CRF stimulates the pituitary gland to release ACTH (adrenocorticotropic hormone). ACTH, as its name implies, stimulates the adrenal gland to produce cortisol.

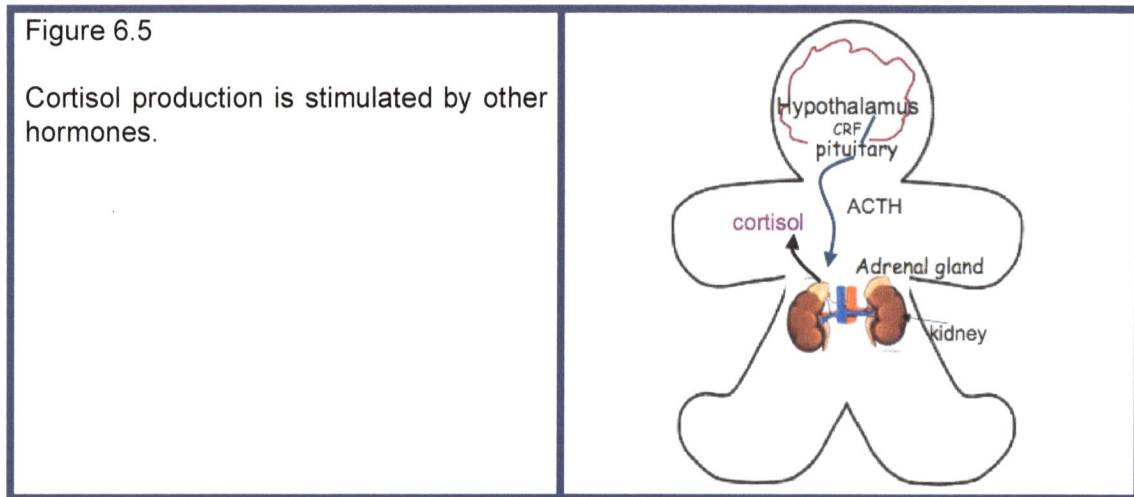

Figure 6.5

Cortisol production is stimulated by other hormones.

Cortisol and adrenaline are both produced in the adrenal glands, but in different locations in the gland. Cortisol is produced in the cortex and epinephrine in the medulla. Epinephrine is produced due to innervation and hence it is rapidly made, as nerve from brain stimulates it production. The production of cortisol is slower. Cortisol's effect on metabolism is slower too. Cortisol stimulates the synthesis of key enzymes involved in glucogeneogenesis. It takes time to make a protein.

6.13 Summary
GB did what Mom said not to do: GB skipped breakfast. Yet, blood glucose did not go low, and GB passed a Calculus exam. The liver made glucose from amino acids. Cortisol stimulated the break-down of some proteins mainly in muscle. It also stimulated the synthesis of enzymes that catalyze the reactions that make glucose in the liver.

6.14 Case study

Health care people say that they "practice medicine." This is a good phrase because it means that they recognize that they do not know everything and that they should learn from their patients. The group of patients described in this case helps to emphasize the importance of gluconeogenesis.

A group of children who have hypoglycemia (low blood sugar) with high keto-acids in the morning
Pagliara et al., J. Clinical. Investigation, 51, 1972, 1440-1449 Hypoalaninemia: a concomitant of ketotic hypoglycemia

Physicians observed that some children have low blood sugar and high keto-acids when they wake up after sleeping. In the paper cited above, 8 of these children were studied and compared with children whose blood sugar remains normal. The children ranged in age from 30 to 56 months. The affected children were all small (growth in the 20th percentile or lower) for their age. Most of the children suffered from seizures, and several had experienced coma.

The children were given glucose tolerance tests. This test is described in Fig. 5.8. Glucose levels during this test were the same within error for the patients and the control group. The glucose tolerance tests shows that the insulin response was normal. Glucose goes into glycogen during this test, and therefore the children are able to make glycogen. In both patient and control children, glucose in the blood went up, indicating that glycogen from the liver was broken down.

Next the investigators gave alanine by intravenous infusion. The glucose levels in the children went up, but not as high as normal.

The final test was to give the children cortisol. In this case, alanine restored glucose levels to normal.

The diagnosis was that in these children, cortisol was low. When cortisol was present, the children's level of alanine went up because cortisone stimulates the break-down of muscle, thereby releasing alanine. The glucose levels went up because cortisone also stimulates the enzymes of gluconeogenesis and alanine was made into glucose.

The children usually "out-grow" this condition, and by age 5 or 6 they produce appropriate levels of cortisone so that gluconeogenesis occurs during short-time fasting.

6.15 Appendix for additional study

The pathways to make something are always different from the pathways to break something down. We see that in glycogen synthesis. The enzymes that make glycogen are different from the enzymes that break glycogen down.

Glycolyis (break down of glucose) and gluconeogenesis (the making of glucose) pathways are unique in that both pathways share some enzymes. But some important enzymes are stimulated or inhibited and this is what ensures that the proper pathway is operating. Figure 6.12 shows the key enzymes that are activated or inhibited.

Starting from alanine, muscle breakdown is stimulated by cortisol. Alanine is transformed into pyruvate by transamination (it gives it amino group to another compound).

Pyruvate kinase is inhibited. High glucogon stimulates the formation of a compound called cyclic AMP, this stimulates an enzyme called protein kinase. Protein kinase puts a phosphate onto pyruvate kinase, and the enzyme becomes inhibited.

Pyruvate goes into the mitochondria where a C is added to it by **pyruvate carboxylase**. This enzyme is stimulated by acetyl CoA. Acetyl CoA is high when fatty acids are being used for fuel. Fatty acids are used for fuel in I/G is low. Fatty acid oxidation supplies ATP, needed for gluconeogenesis.

PEP carboxykinase converts 4 C to 3 C. The synthesis of this enzyme is stimulated by cortisol. Without cortisol present, there is little PEP carboxykinase.

Fructose phosphatase is stimulated by low I/G. It is not directly stimulated, but indirectly; an activator fructose 2.6-bisphosphate. Fructose phosphatase is inhibited by AMP . AMP is high when ATP is low; high AMP, on the other hand, stimulates phosphofrutokinase, an enzyme of glycolysis.

Glucose-6-phosphatase converts glucose-6-phosphate to glucose. This enzyme is in the endoplasmic reticulum. Its synthesis is stimulated by cortisol.

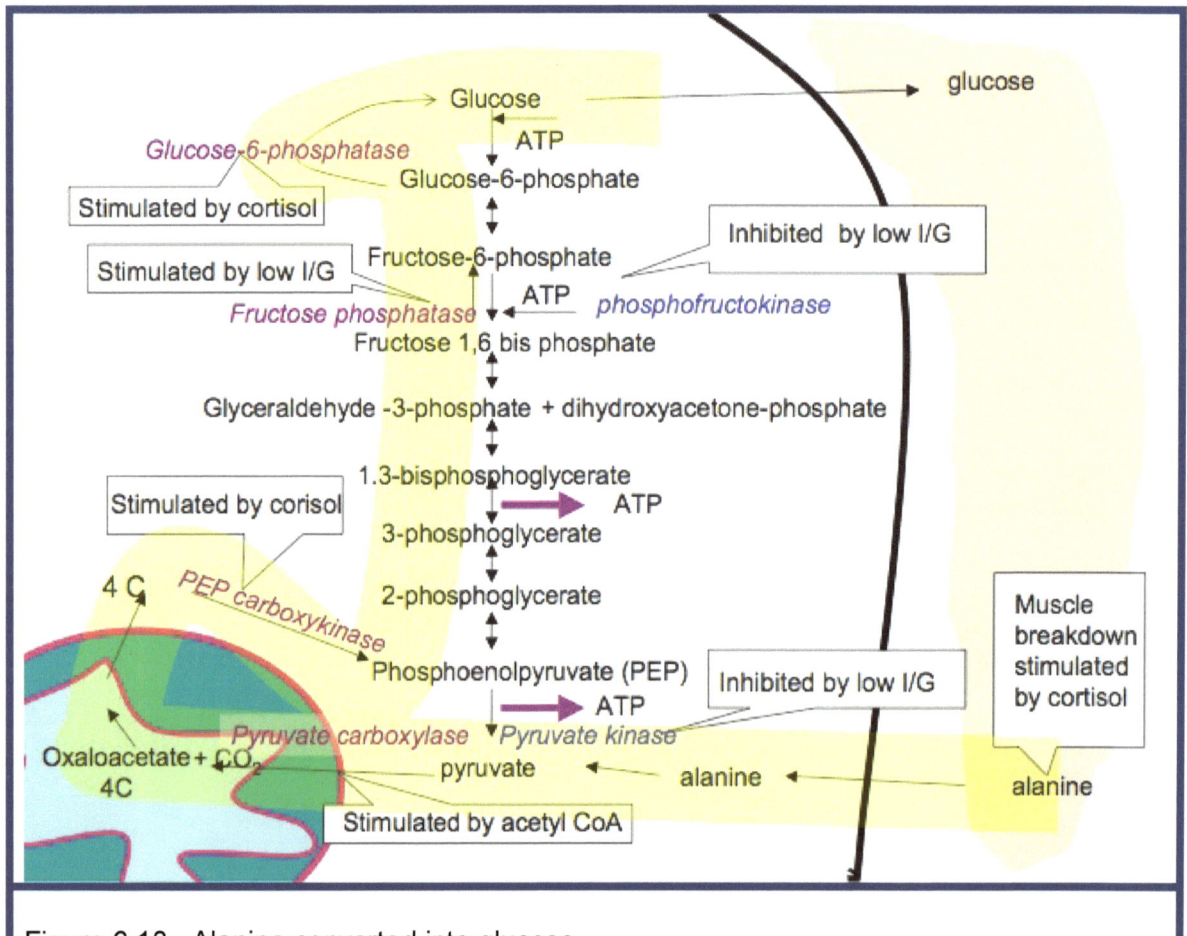

Figure 6.13 Alanine converted into glucose.

The right side (beige) of the figure refers to muscle. The left side shows what is happening in the liver.

7. Making and storing fat and retrieving it to supply energy

7.1 Fat is the major storage form of fuel

Fat is required for human life. In chapter 5 we noted that the amount of glycogen, the storage form of carbohydrates, is limited in the body. You can survive, perhaps, for only about one day on stored glycogen. With fat, you can survive for weeks. Eating more and more will make you fatter and fatter as fat accumulates in the cells of the adipose tissues. Although fat is stored mainly in adipose tissue, most cells that contain mitochondria also have fat globules in them. You may ask why does the body not simply store glycogen – why bother storing fat? It would make studying metabolism easier! But, a pound of fat has about twice the calories as a pound of glycogen. If you have 20 pounds of excess fat, to store the same amount of calories as glycogen would require 40 pounds.

Most tissues can use fat to make ATP. Metabolism of fat always requires O_2 and fatty acids are degraded to form CO_2 in the mitochondria. CO_2 is removed from the body by breathing, and it ultimately goes to the atmosphere.

Two types of cells are notable in that they do not use fat as a fuel. Red blood cells (RBC's) have no mitochondria and consequently RBC'S do not use fat. Brain has mitochondria but it does not use fat for energy. The reason for this is that fat in circulating blood does not cross the specialized capillaries of the brain (these capillaries are called the blood brain barrier). We learned before that brain uses glucose for fuel. However, as we will discuss in this chapter, under long term fasting, the brain switches fuel from glucose to ketoacid compounds. Liver makes ketoacids from fat, and so only under non-feeding conditions, does brain indirectly uses fat.

Fat is triglyceride. It has three fatty acids attached to glycerol. Liver is the main organ for making fat, although the pathway for fatty acid synthesis is present in liver, brain, kidney, mammary gland, adipose tissue and others. Fat is made in the liver from excess carbohydrates, which includes sugar and flour and from excess proteins.

Fat from food also directly contribute to fat stores. Ingested fat goes from the intestine into the lymph system and then into the circulating blood. Ingested fat is carried in the blood in particles called chylomicrons. Many tissues can use the circulating fat, but if these tissues have no need for ATP they do not use fat from the diet and fat is taken into adipose tissue for storage. The transport of fat, and the relationship of fat and cholesterol to manifestations of atherosclerosis (heart disease, stroke), is an important health concern that will be discussed in the next chapter.

7.2. Making fat and retrieving fatty acids from the fat stores

Fat is made when excess food is eaten. Stored fat is used for energy when food is lacking. In Figures 7.1-7.3, GB is used to illustrate three stages of making and using fat.

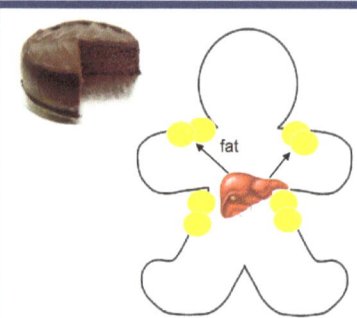	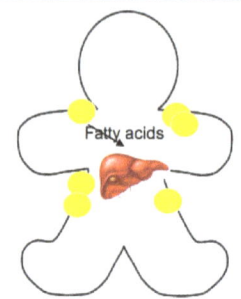	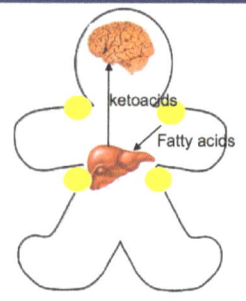
Figure 7.1. Fat synthesis. GB's liver is making fat from carbohydrates. His adipose tissue size is increasing. Insulin is high and glucogon is low.	Figure 7.2. Fat breakdown. Most tissues are using fat for fuel during short-term starvation. Liver is using fat to make ATP, for gluconeogenesis. GB is getting thinner. Insulin is low and glucogon is high.	Figure 7.3. Long-term starvation. The liver is converting fatty acids into ketoacids. Brain and other tissues are using ketoacids for fuel. GB is losing most of his fat. Insulin is low, and glucogon and cortisol are high.

Phase 1. Fat synthesis: AcetylCoA is made into fatty acids in the cytoplasm. Fatty acid synthesis requires NADPH. The "pentose phosphate shunt" pathway supplies NADPH. The pentose phosphate shunt is a simple pathway, but it is involved in diverse other pathways and important diseases (Chapter 9). Glycolysis makes 3 C compounds from glucose and pyruvate dehydrogenase takes 3 C to 2 C, i,e. acetylCoA. Fatty acids are made from acetyl-CoA, and they are assembled into triglycerides (i.e., fat) in the cytoplasm of liver cells.

Phase 2. Fat breakdown: Triglycerides are broken down into fatty acids and glycerol. Fatty acids are bound to the protein albumin when they are transported in the blood. In the tissues using fatty acids for fuel, the fatty acids are broken down to form acetylCoA in mitochondria using the β-oxidation pathway. The acetyl group gets broken down to H_2O and CO_2 using the citric acid cycle and oxidative phosphorylation (Chapter 4). Many ATP molecules are formed.

Phase 3. Ketoacids during starvation: Ketoacids are made from AcetylCoA from fat during long-term starvation. The liver makes ketoacids but does not use ketoacids for fuel. All organs with mitochondria – except the liver – are able to use ketoacids for fuel.

7.3 Phase 1. Fat synthesis

Fat is made in the liver from excess carbohydrates and amino acids. Figure 7.4 gives an overview of what happens when sugar is converted into fatty acid.

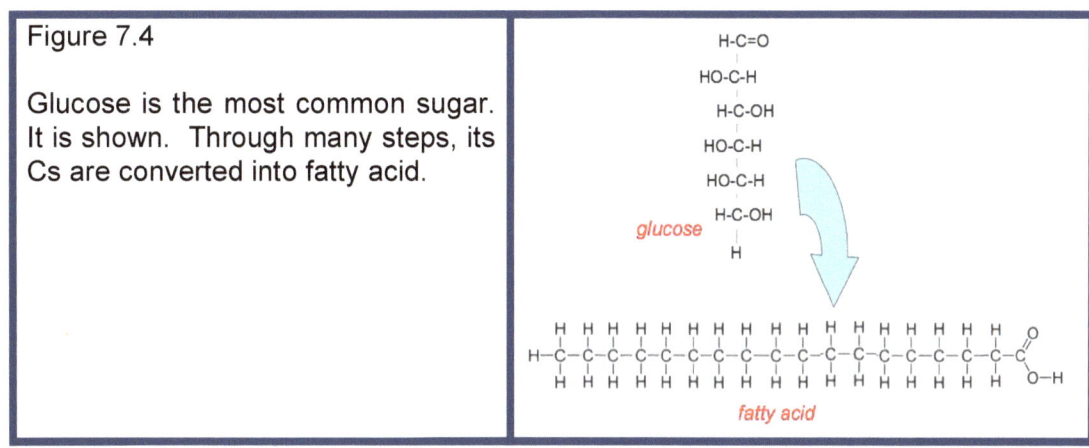

Figure 7.4

Glucose is the most common sugar. It is shown. Through many steps, its Cs are converted into fatty acid.

You notice two differences between glucose and fatty acid. Glucose has equal number of O's and C's. Fatty acids have fewer O's and more H's. Sugars usually have 6 C's whereas fatty acids usually have 16 to 18 C's. So, to make fatty acids, O must be eliminated and the molecule must be made longer.

7.3.1 Carbohydrates can be converted into fatty acids

Here is what we have learned before: carbohydrates get broken to three C compounds in the cytoplasm and then to two C, acetyl CoA, in the mitochondria. In the mitochondria acetyl CoA gets broken down to CO_2 with the formation of ATP. We know in general terms how acetyl CoA break-down in the mitochondria is regulated: when the cell uses up ATP, ADP is formed. ADP stimulates the electron-transport chain and NADH goes to NAD. High NAD stimulates the reactions in the Citric acid cycle that uses up acetyl-CoA. This is shown in Figure 7.5.

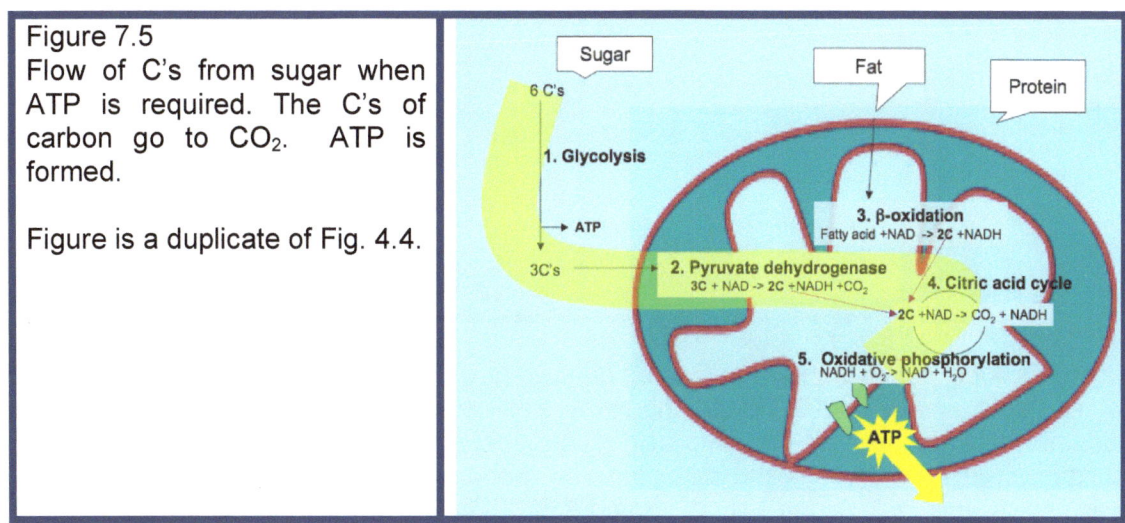

Figure 7.5
Flow of C's from sugar when ATP is required. The C's of carbon go to CO_2. ATP is formed.

Figure is a duplicate of Fig. 4.4.

When more acetyl-CoA is made than is needed to make ATP (when you are eating excess carbohydrate), liver converts acetylCoA into fatty acid. Figure 7.6 shows the pathways going from glucose to fatty acid.

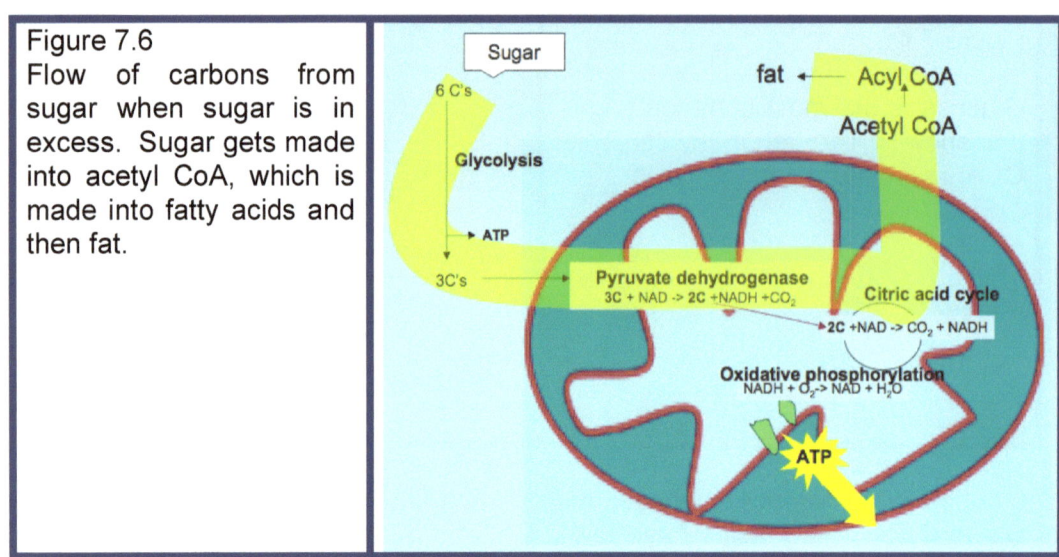

Figure 7.6
Flow of carbons from sugar when sugar is in excess. Sugar gets made into acetyl CoA, which is made into fatty acids and then fat.

In this picture, you see that glucose gets chopped into three C compound, pyruvate, by the glycolysis pathway in the cytoplasm. Then CO_2 is removed from pyruvate and the two C compound, acetyl CoA is formed in the mitochondria. The acetyl CoA leaves the mitochondria and it is made into acyl CoA, and then assembled into triglyceride, i.e. fat.

Acetyl CoA does not directly leave the mitochondria, however. Here is a more expanded view of fatty acid synthesis for what happens to the C's.

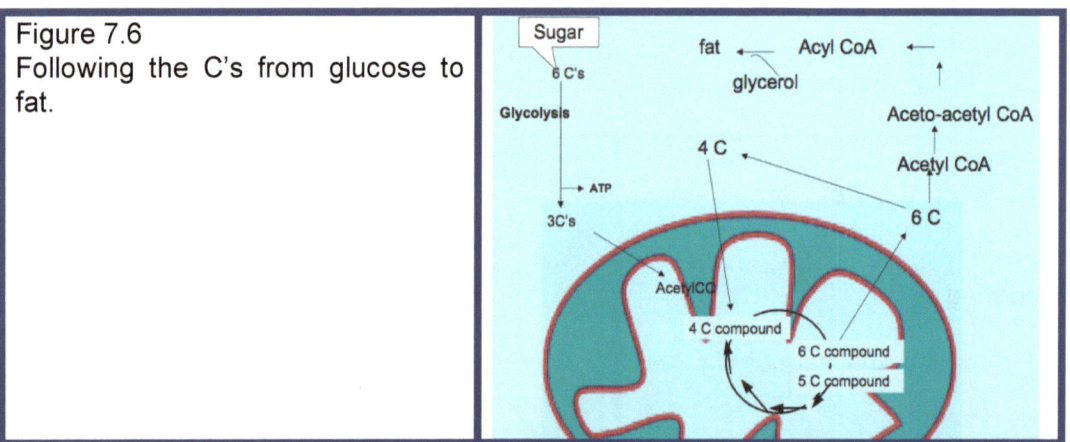

Figure 7.6
Following the C's from glucose to fat.

Acetyl CoA combines with a four C compound to form a six C compound; this compound is citric acid, and in the TCA cycle, the two C's get converted to CO_2. When ATP is not required, the reactions of the citric acid cycle slow down, and citric acid concentration builds up. It then crosses the mitochondrial membrane. The six C compound, citric acid, splits into four C and two C compounds. The two C compound is the familiar compound, acetyl CoA. The 4 C compound goes back into the mitochondria, and is part of the citric acid cycle.

Acetyl CoA hooks onto another acetyl CoA to form a four C compound, acetoacetyl CoA.

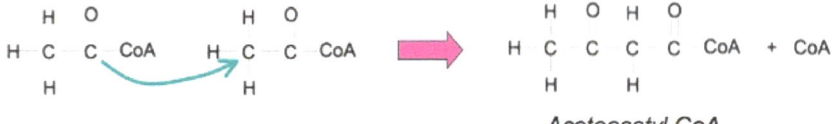

Acetoacetyl CoA

Acetoacetyl CoA is now 4 C's long. It still contains an oxygen atom that must be gotten rid of. NADPH adds H's to it, and H_2O is removed in a series of steps. NADPH is like NADH, except that NADPH has an extra phosphate group.

Another acetyl CoA adds on to the four C compound, and the O atom is removed and H's added. We now have a six C compound. The steps are repeated until 16 or 18 C's are attached. The final product is 16 or 18 C fatty acid in the form of CoA, also called acyl CoA.

The fatty acids are attached to glycerol, and the final product, fat, is obtained.

7.3.2 NADPH is supplied by the pentose phosphate shunt

The C's for fat synthesis come from glucose. It turns out that glucose also supplies the extra H's required to make fat by supplying NADPH. NADPH is made in a pathway called the **pentose phosphate shunt**. The name "pentose phosphate shunt" arises because pentose phosphate is a product, and "shunt" is used because this pathway shunts C's from the glycolytic pathway. (Some textbooks call this pathway the "hexose monophosphate pathway." Glucose 6-phosphate, a hexose monophosphate, is the starting material of this pathway, hence this name). NADPH is like NADH but it has a phosphate attached to it. Enzymes that use NADPH cannot use NADH and vice versa. So the synthesis of fat is dependent upon the presence of NADPH.

The enzymes for this pathway are located in the cytoplasm of all cells. This makes sense because NADPH is used to make fat, and fat synthesis is also in the cyotoplasm.

The cell uses the pentose phosphate shunt to make NADPH and ribose-5-P, a five C sugar. The production of which product depends upon the needs of the cell. 5 C sugars are used in the making of DNA and ATP, and then much ribose-5-P is used. When fat synthesis is going on, the important metabolite of the pentose phosphate shunt is NADP. The NADPH comes from the pentose shunt is involved in fat synthesis in the liver as seen in Figure 7.7. In Chapter 9 we will talk about the use of the pentose phosphate shunt in repair of damaged proteins.

Figure 7.7.	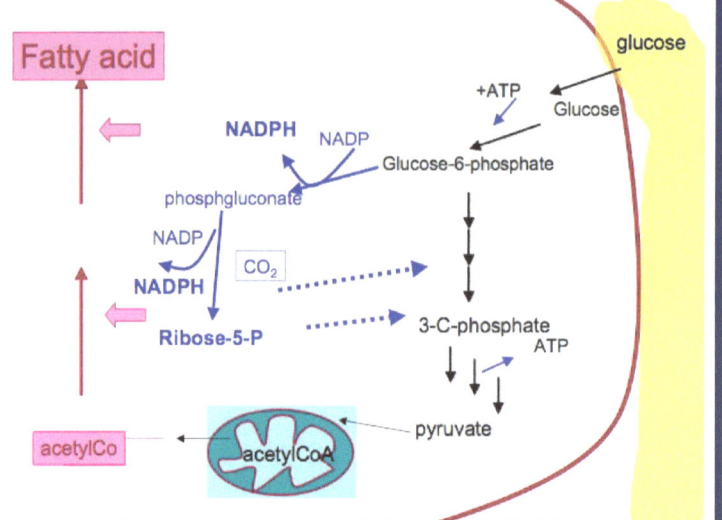
Glucose reacts with NADP to form phosphogluconate and NADPH. NADPH gives H's to make fat. Phosphogluconate loses CO_2 to form a 5C sugar, called ribose-5-P. The ribose sugar rearranges to form 3 C compounds and these ultimately make pyruvate.	

So, both the C's and H's of fat come from sugar. Notice that the making of sugar is not 100% efficient in saving C's. One C is lost in the pentose phosphate shunt. And a C is also lost in going from pyruvate to acetyl CoA. No process is 100 % efficient in the body. The making of fat from glucose is still advantageous because when fat is broken down so many ATP molecules are formed.

7.4 Phase 2. Fat mobilization and use

Fat from the adipose is used to make ATP in most tissues when glucose in the blood is low.

Figure 7.8 gives an overview of fat mobilization. Triglyceride, fat is stored in the adipose tissue. When insulin is low and glucogon and adrenaline is high – i.e. when a person is not eating -- a protein called lipase is activated.

Figure 7.8	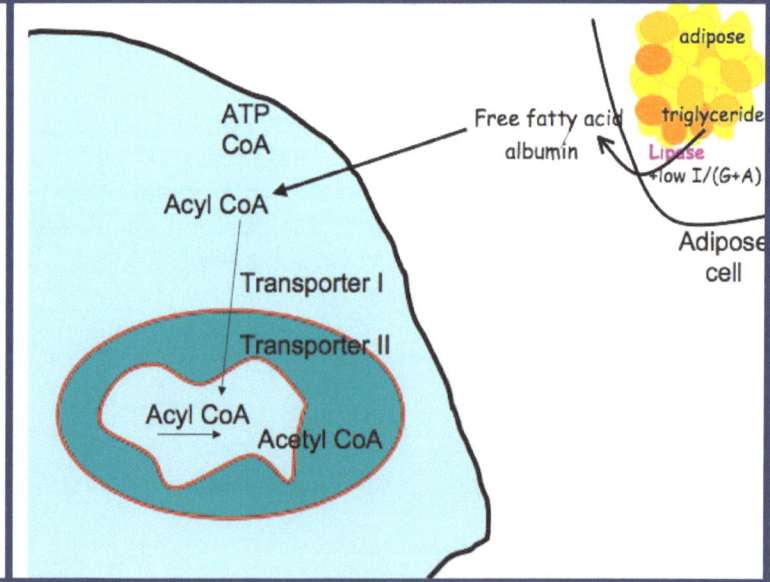
Fat is released from the adipose tissue when insulin is low and glucogon and adrenaline is high. The fat gets broken into free fatty acid by an enzyme called lipase. The fat binds to albumin in the blood. The free fatty acid gets taken in the cells that use fat. A CoA gets put on. The acyl CoA gets transported into the mitochondria by transporter molecules. Acyl CoA gets broken down to acetyl CoA. Acetyl CoA gets broken down to CO_2 and ATP is formed.	

Fat is hydrolyzed to form fatty acids and transported bound to the protein albumin. When you are fasting, fatty acid in the blood increases. In blood work from your doctor's office, this is called FFA, free fatty acid.

Figure 7.9. Albumin

Albumin is a protein in the blood serum. It binds fatty acids strongly; in the picture the green molecules are fatty acids and the blue is the polypeptide chain of albumin; many fatty acids are bound to one albumin molecule. Albumin transports fatty acids from adipose to cells that use fat for energy. Most cells use fatty acids from albumin, but the brain does not, since fatty acids bound to albumin do not pass through the blood brain barrier. Albumin is also shown in Fig. 2.2.

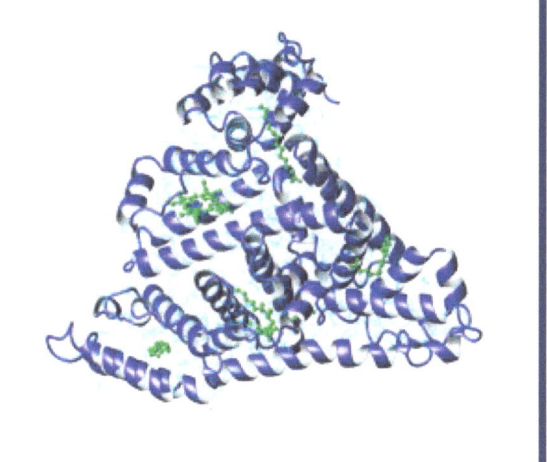

Fatty acid gets taken into a cell. Fatty acid then gets broken down to acetyl CoA, and then to CO_2 in the mitochondria. The steps are given in Chapter 4. Many molecules of ATP are formed.

In some tissues, fat oxidation is occurring at all times. The heart primarily uses fatty acids for fuel. So while fat may be being made in the liver, the heart is oxidizing fat to CO_2 and H_2O.

7.5 Phase 3. Long term fasting and the use of ketoacids.

We are now going back to our patient, GB. We are considering his metabolism under starvation conditions. He has not eaten for several days.

In short-term fasting, proteins from muscle and other tissue are converted into glucose by the liver and used by the brain. In long-term starvation, the body has the means to turn down the use of protein and to turn up the use of fat. It does it by making ketoacids from acetyl CoA. This is good! The metabolism of fat gives more calories than protein; this is to say fat metabolism produces more ATP. Because proteins are used for important functions in the body, it is beneficial to spare the use of proteins for fuel.

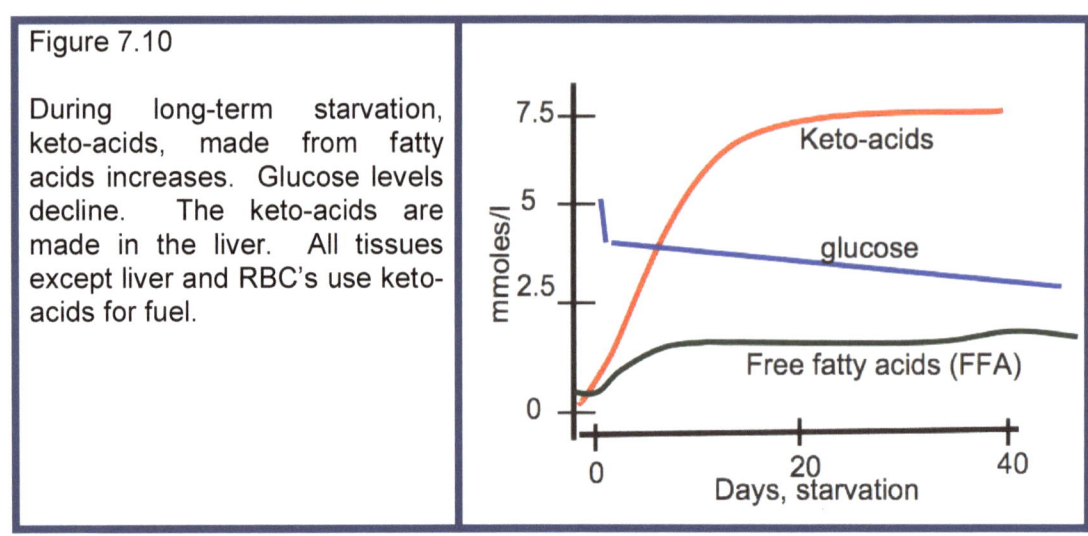

Figure 7.10

During long-term starvation, keto-acids, made from fatty acids increases. Glucose levels decline. The keto-acids are made in the liver. All tissues except liver and RBC's use keto-acids for fuel.

During long-term starvation, fatty acids are transported to the liver, and acetyl CoA builds up. The two ketoacids that are produced by the liver are acetylacetic acid and β-hydroxybutyric acid, shown here[1]:

$$\underset{\text{acetylacetate}}{\text{H}_3\text{C}-\text{CO}-\text{CH}_2-\text{COOH}} \qquad \underset{\beta\text{-hydroxybutyrate}}{\text{H}_3\text{C}-\text{CHOH}-\text{CH}_2-\text{COOH}}$$

Ketoacids are made in the mitochondria of the <u>liver only</u>.[2] Cortisol stimulates the enzymes that make ketoacids in the liver. After synthesis, acetoacetate and β–hydroxybutyrate go into the blood stream. Most tissues, including heart, skeletal muscle and brain use them for fuel. Liver does not use them for fuel because the enzymes to break them down are not found in the liver. RBC's do not use them for fuel, because they are metabolized to CO_2 and O_2 in mitochondria, and RBC's do not have mitochondria.

The enzymes that break down ketoacids in tissues other than liver increase during starvation. These enzymes are stimulated by cortisol. The ketoacids get broken down to acetyl CoA. Acetyl CoA gets broken down to CO_2 in the citric acid cycle and ATP is made by oxidative phosphorylation.

Notice that the liver is again the "good guy"; it makes keto-acids for use in other tissues but it itself does not use them. The production of keto-acids reduces the brains reliance on sugar, which comes from protein during starvation. If you turn back to Figure 6.2, you notice that the amount of glucose made by the liver decreases during long-term fasting. The brain is now using keto-acids for fuel, and so less glucose is needed for the brain to

---

[1] Many text books call these compounds "ketone bodies". Acetylacetate is a keto-acid and β-hydroxybutyrate is a hydroxy acid. Since these two acids interconvert we shall lump both into the term "keto-acids" for simplification. We do not use the word "body", since this is not a term used in organic chemistry.

[2] There is an exception. A few amino acids are converted to keto-acids in muscle.

survive. Since glucose is made from protein, the use of keto-acids for fuel spares the use of protein.

To emphasize, the brain uses glucose as its main fuel, but during starvation it relies upon the use of acetylacetate and β-hydroxybutyrate, the ketoacids. These are 4 C compounds made from fat using acetyl CoA. During this time, the enzymes of the brain also change. Transporters for the ketoacids appear, and the enzymes to break-down ketoacids into acetylCoA appear. Even though the metabolism of the brain has changed, it retains its cognitive functions.

7.6 An additional pathway: Very long chain fatty acids

The fat that we and most animals and plants store is made from 16 and 18 C's fatty acids. But we eat many things and a small portion of the fat that we eat has more than 18 C's. There are enzymes in the lyzosome that have a specialized way to process very long chain fatty acids.

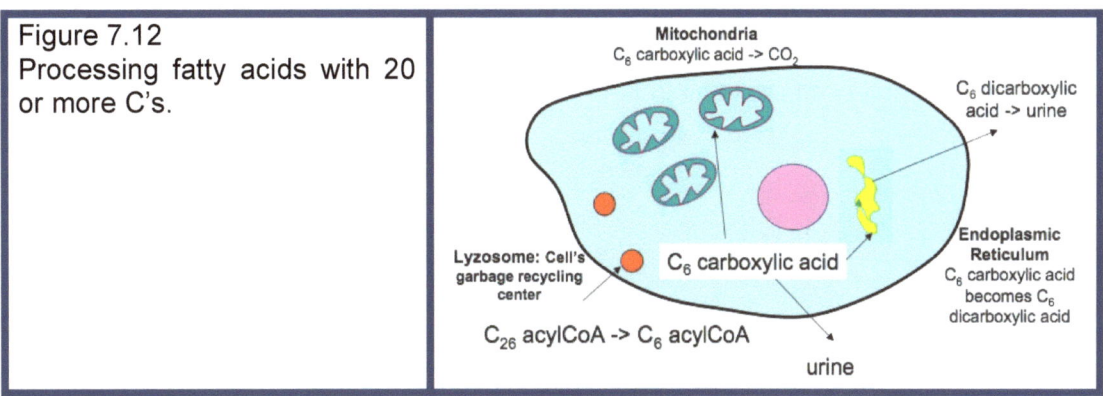

Figure 7.12
Processing fatty acids with 20 or more C's.

The long chain fatty acids are broken down to acetyl CoA and six C acyl CoA. The six C acyl CoA can lose the CoA, and six C carboxylic acid is lost to the blood plasma, and excreted into the urine. Some of the six C acyl carboxylic acid is converted by enzymes in the endoplasmic reticulum to make it have two carboxyl groups on it – one on each end. This compound, a dicarboxylic acid, is excreted into the urine.

The net effect of the enzymes of the lyzosome and the endoplasmic reticulum is called "detoxification". These enzymes act to change many substances that we eat. The lyzosome breaks the substance down, and the endoplasmic reticulum puts carboxyl or sugar groups on the compound to make it more soluble. Then these substances go into the blood stream, and they are excreted in the urine.

Enzymes within the lyzosomes break down long chain fatty acids and other fatty acid compounds with unusual composition. When an enzyme is defective in the lyzosomes, these unusual fatty acids and fat accumulate and cause havoc to the health of the patient.

7.7 Importance of unsaturated fatty acids

Many of diseases of lyzosomes involve neurological symptoms. Lipids form the core of membranes. You remember that K^+ salt is inside cells and Na^+ salt is outside, and that this is essential for nerve function. When the lipids are not of normal composition, this salt distribution across the membrane is disrupted. Diseases of lyzosomes include Tay-Sachs, Pompe, and Gaucher diseases.

The reason that a defect in the metabolism of fatty acids causes problems in processes involving membranes is that membranes are composed of fat-like substances. One of the major components of membranes is lecithin (Chapter 3). Biological membranes are composed of lecithin plus many other compounds similar to lecithin. Instead of the "choline" part, there may be a compound resembling an amino acid or sugar. When the head group is sugar, the compound is called a glycolipid. Glycolipids are found in high amounts in nerve cells. Membranes have different lipids within them. Unsaturated lipids are fluid, and they keep the center, hydrophobic part, flexible. We cannot make lipids that have many unsaturated double bonds, and we must get them from our diet.[3] Some dieticians recommend eating fish oils, high in unsaturated fatty acids, to ensure that we get enough unsaturated fatty acids.

7.8 Concluding comments

Excess dietary carbohydrate and protein are converted into fat for storage. During long-term starvation, fat is converted into keto-acids. The brain uses keto-acids for fuel.

---

[3] Unsaturated fatty acids are also precursors for prostaglandins, hormones that are important in immunity.

8. Fat and cholesterol transport

8.1 Fat and cholesterol are transported in specialized particles

Sugars and amino acids dissolve in water. To transport glucose and amino acids from the liver to another tissue, the substance dissolves in the water of blood, and the heart pumps the blood to all tissues. Fat does not dissolve in water, as you know if you try to dissolve cooking oil in water. Fat is transported in the blood, but the body needs a different system to get fat into the blood. Fat is incorporated in specialized particles in the blood called **lipoproteins**. Lipoproteins are small particles in blood that contain protein, fat and cholesterol.

Some fat comes from the diet and this fat is transported in the blood using one kind of lipoprotein, called **chylomicrons**. Other fats are made in the liver when excess sugar or protein is eaten. Another group of lipoproteins transport this fat. The important lipoprotein in this group is called low-density lipoprotein, or **LDL**. Some of the proteins in chylomicrons and LDL are the same. Finally, there is a particle called high-density lipoprotein, or **HDL**, aids in transfer of the proteins between the particles and in removing cholesterol from tissues.

All lipoproteins contain cholesterol. Hence, we need to talk about cholesterol and fat together. This chapter will describe how fat and cholesterol is transported from the intestine from food and between organs. As always, we are describing what happens in humans – the way that fat and cholesterol are transported is quite different in other animals.

The transport of fat and cholesterol in the blood has major health considerations. People who have high amounts of LDL are more likely to have cardiovascular diseases such as heart attack or stroke. People who have high amounts of HDL have lower risk for these diseases. When your doctor tells how much cholesterol is in your blood, you will be told that LDL is "lousy" or "bad" cholesterol. HDL is "healthy" or "good" cholesterol. The doctor may tell you that if the ratio of LDL to HDL is low, that this is a healthy indication.

8.2 Cholesterol: friend or foe?

Most people are aware that high cholesterol in the blood can contribute to heart attacks and strokes. We talk about our cholesterol levels at parties. Cholesterol seems to be a bad guy! But is it?

What is cholesterol? The structure of cholesterol is shown below. Remember that whenever there is a bend in the structure, the bend represents a C, with associated H's. You see that cholesterol is mostly made up of C's and H's. Since it is made up of mostly C's and H's it is hydrophobic and does not dissolve in water.

Cholesterol

Our bodies make cholesterol. Liver synthesizes most of the body's cholesterol, but all cells that have mitochondria (that basically means all cells except red blood cells) are able to make cholesterol. Cholesterol is made from acetyl (2 carbon) groups.

We also get cholesterol from animal products in diet. Cholesterol is high in animal fat and in dairy foods and eggs. Dairy products and egg yolks are foods that are intended to nourish the young of mammals and birds. The enzymes that make cholesterol are not always developed in the young. It makes sense that the food given to the young would have cholesterol. In fact, some pediatricians recommend that children be given whole milk, which contains cholesterol, rather than skim milk, to drink until they are about five years old. By this time, the child's liver enzymes are developed to make enough to supply the needs of cholesterol.

We do not get cholesterol from plant foods since plants do not make cholesterol. Plants have related molecules (called sitosterol and lanosterol).

We absolutely require cholesterol. No person in the world is living that is known to have no cholesterol – this would not be compatible with human life. There are very rare diseases in which the cholesterol transport from the liver to other tissues is impaired. These patients are very sick.

Cholesterol has important functions in our body:

1. Cholesterol is found in membranes that surround the cell. During development of a baby, the nerves in the brain get covered with membranes called the myelin sheath. Myelin sheath is composed of layers of membranes that are composed of mainly a glycolipid and cholesterol. If a child does not have enough cholesterol, the brain will not develop normally. For the most part, cholesterol is not found in membranes inside of the cell. For instance, mitochondrial membranes do not have cholesterol.
2. Cholesterol is needed to transport fat in the blood stream. All types of lipoproteins contain cholesterol.
3. Cholesterol is used to form vitamin D. Vitamin D regulates calcium levels in the body. Vitamin D is made in our skin in response to light; hence cells in the skin makes it when we are outside in the sunshine. Vitamin D stimulates pumps for Ca^{++} absorption in the intestine. In the kidney, Ca^{++} is lost, but vitamin D stimulates pumps to take Ca^{++} back into the blood. Without vitamin D, therefore, not enough Ca is absorbed from the diet, plus, Ca^{++} in the blood is lost in the urine.
4. The precursor to make cholesterol is also used to make coenzyme Q. Coenzyme Q is found in mitochondria. Mitochondria need coenzyme Q in order to use oxygen and make ATP.
5. Cholesterol is a precursor for bile acids. Bile acids aid in the digestion of fat.

6. Cholesterol is used to make the steroid hormones. Steroid hormones include the sex hormones. Testosterone in males and estrogen in females regulate sex characteristics. Another steroid hormone is cortisol. This hormone is one of many that regulate metabolism.

And this final interesting fact about cholesterol: although we make it and get it from our diet, and we use it in important ways, we do not get calories from it. It is made from 2 C units using enzymes in our cells, but we do not have the enzymes to break it down to acetyl CoA. Consequently, it is not converted to CO_2 and H_2O in the mitochondria. And mitochondria make no ATP from it – no energy, i.e. calories, for the cell.

So right now we have a gigantic idea. Cholesterol is good – we absolutely need it! And we don't get calories from it! Why not eat a lot of cholesterol and stay healthy and slim? The story is more complicated. Too much cholesterol causes many problems. To understand why, we need to know how cholesterol is transported in the body and how the body gets rid of excess cholesterol.

8.3 Fat and cholesterol get into the body in the intestine

Figure 8.1 shows a meal that is high in cholesterol, cholesterol esters and fat. You remember that fat is triglyceride, composed of three fatty acids that are attached to the three OH groups of the glycerol molecule. Cholesterol has one OH (hydroxy) group and a fatty acid can also attach to fatty acid. Then it is called cholesterol ester. Diet will contain both cholesterol esters and cholesterol. Figure 8.1 shows what happens to the fat and cholesterol after a meal.

Figure 8.1.

Step 1. Fat and cholesterol from the diet gets emulsified by bile acids in the intestine. Bile acids are themselves made from cholesterol.
Step 2. Fat and cholesterol gets packaged into chylomicrons. The bile acids are recyled by being taken up again by the intestine and returned to the gall bladder. Some are lost in the feces.
Step 3. Chylomicrons pass into the lymph system and then into the blood.
Step 4. Adipose (fat tissue) and other tissues take the triglyceride from the chylomicrons. The chylomicron particle gradually becomes smaller, until it is the chylomicron remnant, rich in cholesterol.
Step 5. The liver takes in the remnant.

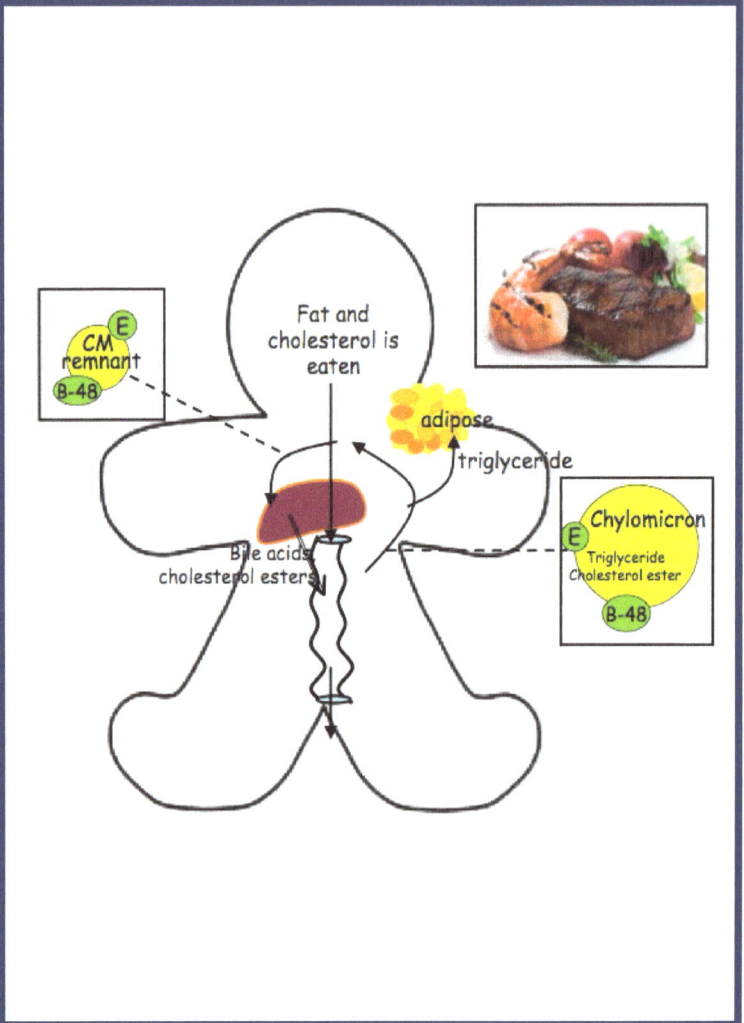

Step 1. When we eat fat, cholesterol and cholesterol esters these water insoluble molecules get "emulsified" by bile acids. This is the same process that cleans clothes in the washing machine. The soap in the washing machine or the bile acids in the intestine break up globules of fat to smaller particles. One of the most common bile acid is cholic acid that itself is made from cholesterol. This is the structure of cholic acid.

You see that it looks like cholesterol but has more OH groups on it. The process of emulsification occurs in the intestine. Bile acids, made from cholesterol by the liver, are stored in the gall bladder. They are secreted into the intestine, and they break up fat into particles that are suspended in water. An analogous process breaks up fat in your frying pan when you clean it with dishwashing detergent.

Step 2. The intestine transfers fat and cholesterol across the intestinal wall. In cells called enterocytes, fat and cholesterol are assembled into a particle called the chylomicron. Chylomicrons contain fat, cholesterol and cholesterol esters and they are held together by specialized proteins called apoproteins. These proteins are named apoA, apoB, apoC and apoE (Figure 8.2).

Some of the bile acid molecules are reabsorbed to be used again, and some are lost in the feces. The loss of bile acids during digestion results in less cholesterol in the body. This is an important way to reduce the amount of cholesterol in the body.

Step 3. The chylomicron goes from the enterocyte into the lymph system. From the lymph it goes to the subclavian vein, where the fat goes into the general blood circulation.[4] Fat soluble vitamins, such as vitamin A and D, also enter the body through this system. They get distributed to the various tissues, initially by-passing the enzymes in the liver that would remove them by "detoxification" described briefly in the last chapter.

Figure 8.2	
Fat and cholesterol from the diet gets packaged into particles that get transferred to the left subclavian vein. This vein connects eventually to the superior vena cava vein, which brings blood to the heart. The heart pumps the blood into the general circulation. (Doctors always refer to left and right relative to the patient. So although the left subclavian vein on the picture is on the right, it would be on the left on the patient.)	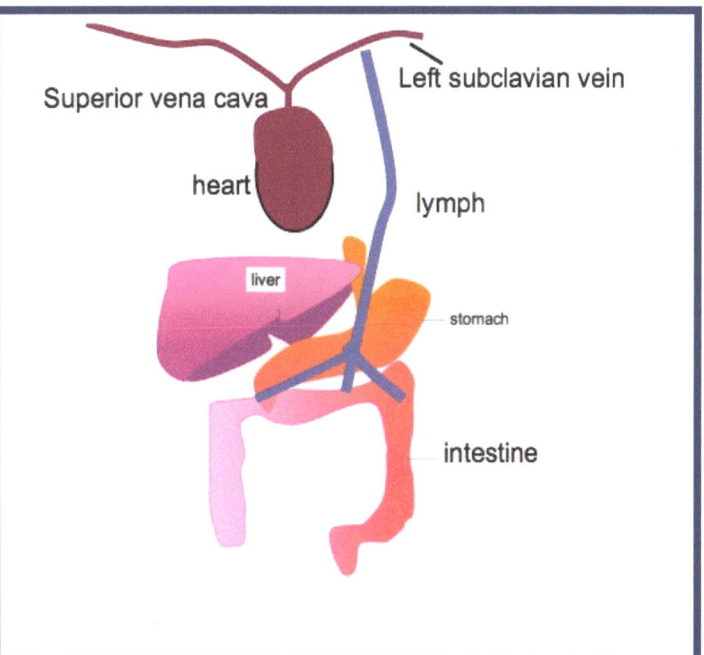

Step 4. After eating a big meal of fat, your blood plasma appears milky from chylomicrons. The adipose cells (i.e. our fat) recognize the proteins E and B-48 on the chylomicrons, and the chylomicrons transiently bind to the cells. During this process the triglyceride within the chylomicron is transferred to adipose and other tissues. Gradually,

---

4 You notice that the treatment of fat by digestion is quite different from protein and carbohydrates. Proteins are broken down to amino acids and carbohydrates are broken to single sugars in the intestine. The portal vein transports these to the liver. The liver transforms the sugars and amino acids, and then they get into the general circulation.

over a period of hours, the chylomicrons become depleted of fat, and then the particle is called chylomicron remnant.

Figure 8.3 Proteins of chylomicrons are shown as magenta spheres, phospholipids are represented by blue circles with tails. Triglycerides and cholesterol are represented by yellow and orange, respectively. During circulation triglycerides are transferred to adipose tissue (Step 4). The particle loses apoC. It is now called chylomicron remnant.	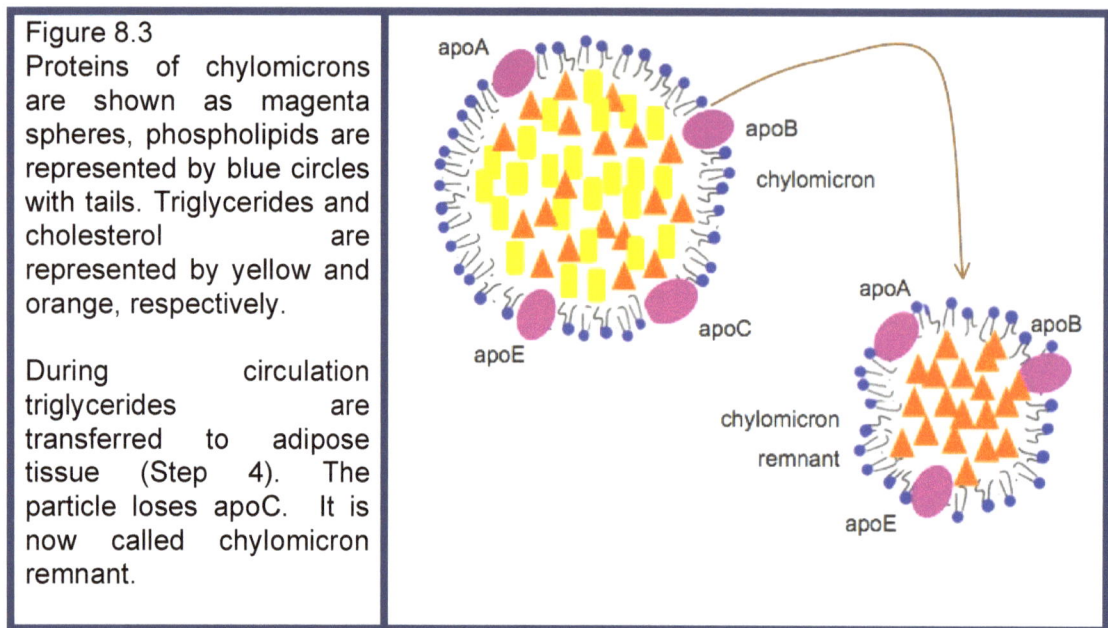

Step 5. The remnant retains most of the cholesterol. The liver recognizes the proteins on the chylomicron particle and it engulfs it (this is called endocytosis), and the cholesterol from the diet becomes part of the pool of cholesterol in the liver.

If you have ever had your blood cholesterol tested, you will remember that you needed to fast before the test. The reason for fasting is to test cholesterol made in your body and not the transient high levels of cholesterol due to a Big Mac you might have just eaten. So, testing is carried out after all the chylomicrons arising from eating have disappeared from circulation. This takes several hours, and usually you are instructed not to eat over night.

8. 4. Plants have sterols but the intestine excretes them.

Plants have sterols that are related to cholesterol but are not exactly the same. Fat and sterols from plants are emulsified by the intestine, and transported across the intestine. The fats from plants become part of the chylomicron, and the triglycerides get stored in the adipose tissue. But plant sterols are immediately transported back out into the intestine and they are excreted in the feces. They are transported back into the intestine by proteins called ABC proteins. This process involves ATP and a variety of proteins: ABC stands for ATP Binding Cassette. Because the ABC proteins transport plant sterols back into the intestine, plants do not contribute to the body's pool of cholesterol (Figure 8.4).

Figure 8.4	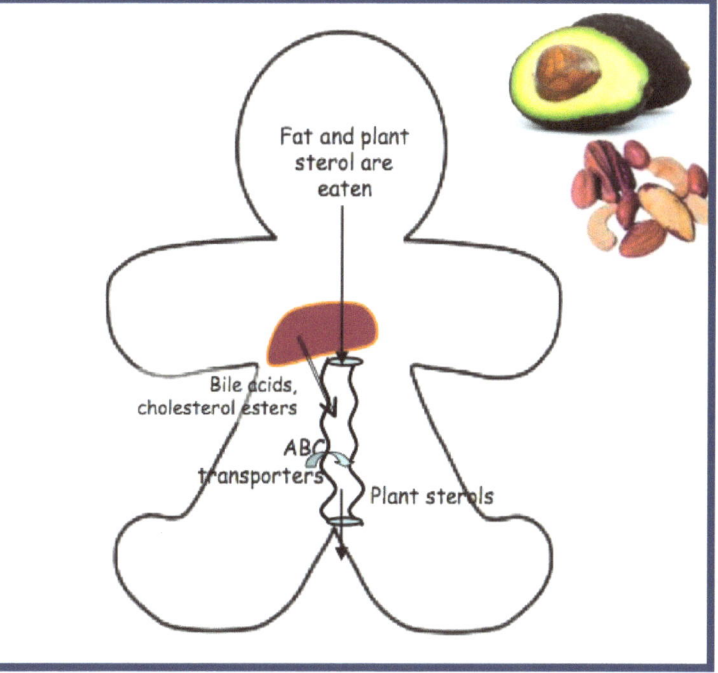
Fate of plant sterols. Plant fats are emulsified just as animal fats are. The plant sterols get taken in the intestine wall, but then they are transported back across the intestine wall by the ABC transporters. The plant sterols are excreted in the feces. Plant fat gets made into chylomicrons.	

8.5 Fat and cholesterol made in the liver are transported by lipoproteins called LDL and VLDL

You know that when you eat too many sweets your adipose tissue increases -- you get fat. Triglycerides are made mainly in the liver. We now come to how triglycerides and cholesterol that are made in the liver are transported to other tissues. Like fat from food that is transported on a lipoprotein particle (namely the chylomicron), fat made in the liver is exported from the liver by a lipoprotein particle. The particle is Very Low Density Lipoprotein, or **VLDL**. It is low density because it is mainly composed of fat and fat floats to the top. (The reason that cream floats to the top of milk is the same: cream is rich in lipoproteins).

VLDL circulates through the blood and gradually triglycerides are removed from it as fat goes into adipose tissue.   It gradually gets smaller and smaller and finally becomes a particle called low-density lipoprotein, or LDL. Since, triglyceride has been removed, the cholesterol in LDL is high relative to the amount of triglyceride.

For the liver to make VLDL, cholesterol is required.   When the liver is making fat, it also makes more cholesterol in order to make VLDL. This is why if you have high cholesterol and are overweight from eating too much carbohydrates and proteins, your physician may recommend that you lose weight. When you are no longer making fat from sugar, you will also not be making so much cholesterol.

Figure 8.5	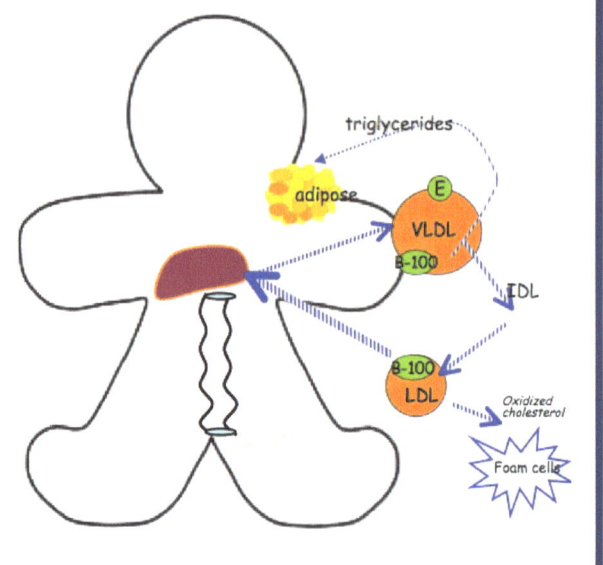
VLDL particles carry triglycerides and cholesterol to adipose and to other tissues. As the triglyceride is depleted, the particle gets smaller (indicated by IDL, intermediate density lipoprotein) and finally becomes LDL, low-density lipoprotein. LDL is rich in cholesterol. Some of the cholesterol can get oxidized. These LDL particles are taken into scavenger cells, on the vascular cells. They form foam cells and lead to atherosclerosis (heart disease and stroke). The liver takes in most LDL particles.	

8.5.1. Why are LDL and VLDL called the "lousy" and "very lousy" lipoproteins?

LDL stands for "low density lipoprotein", but you can also consider that it as "lousy" lipoprotein. This is because it contains the "bad" cholesterol. The reason it is called bad is that there is a correlation between high levels of LDL and vascular diseases. Most doctors consider that if you have high levels of these lousy LDL's you are at increased risk for heart attack and stroke, and the doctor will recommend medicine to reduce the levels of LDL.

High levels of LDL's lead to the formation of plaque, and foam cells in the arteries. As cholesterol circulates through O_2 – rich blood, some of the cholesterol reacts with O_2. The by-product formed – oxy-cholesterol – is thought to trigger an immune response. This makes foam cells grow. Blood is no longer able to flow through the artery.

8.5.2. HDL- the "Happy" or "Healthy" lipoprotein

In rough terms, the function of VLDL is to move triglycerides and cholesterol to adipose and other tissues. There is another particle in the blood whose function is to move cholesterol from tissues to the liver. HDL, standing for "high-density lipoprotein", is the transport particle. In simple terms, its function is to remove cholesterol from the outlying tissues and deliver it to the liver. It has a protein, called apoA. The liver recognizes the apo A protein, and it endocytoses HDL, thereby removing cholesterol from the circulation. In the liver the cholesterol from HDL becomes part of the cholesterol pool in the liver.

Figure 8.6	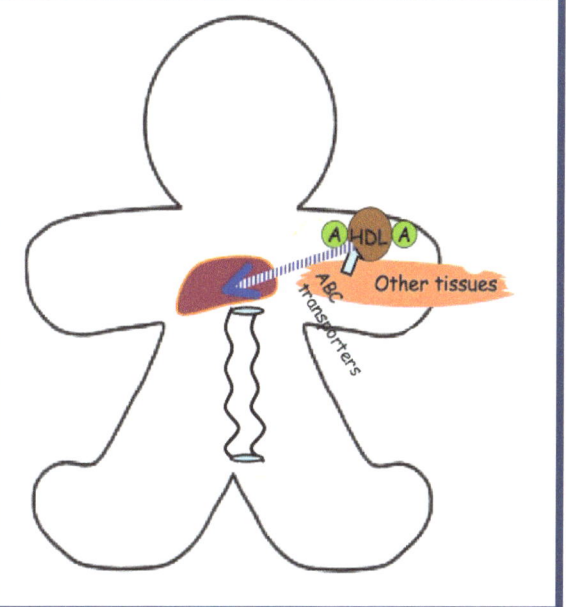
HDL takes cholesterol from outlying tissues and brings it to the liver. Liver makes most of the body's cholesterol. When cholesterol and cholesterol esters get high within the liver, the enzymes that are needed to produce cholesterol are reduced, and the overall liver production of cholesterol goes down. When cholesterol levels within the liver are low, then the enzymes that make cholesterol go up.	

It seems that HDL also serves to transfer the apoproteins between the lipoproteins. There are some families that have very high cholesterol, and have no incidence of atherosclerosis or heart disease. But, for most people, high LDL and low HDL is an indication of likelihood of disease, but exceptions indicate that we do not know the whole story.

8.6. How to keep LDL ("lousy" cholesterol) low and HDL, ("healthy" lipoprotein) high

If cholesterol from LDL in the blood is too high, there is an increase risk of heart disease and stroke, as we mentioned before. So, based upon our knowledge of cholesterol transport what are we to do?

An obvious first step is to lower the amount of cholesterol that we eat. Plants do not contain cholesterol and a diet high in plants will aid in reducing cholesterol.

Another recommendation for people who are overweight is to decrease the intake of food, especially carbohydrates. Extra carbohydrates are converted into triglyceride (fat) in the liver. This fat is transported in the LDL particles to other tissue. For LDL particles to be formed, cholesterol is needed, and therefore the liver makes cholesterol for this purpose

Another approach is to get rid of cholesterol already in the body. How can we do this? Products of cholesterol are the bile acids. Some of the bile acids are reabsorbed in the intestine, but the rest are excreted in the feces. There are resins that hinder the reabsorption of cholesterol and bile acids by the intestine. Such compounds occur naturally in some foods. Oats contain a substance that prevents reabsorption of the cholic acids. Cereals containing oat grain, such as oatmeal and oat containing cereals, such as Cheerios, are advertised as being "heart healthy", Indeed, clinical studies showed that eating such food helps reduce cholesterol levels.

A breakfast that may aid in reducing cholesterol is shown on Figure 8.7. Oatmeal, bananas and peanuts contain no cholesterol, and oatmeal helps to reduce cholesterol. Oats contain a substance that reduces the reabsorption of cholesterol and bile acids back from the intestine back to the liver.

Figure 8.7

A low-cholesterol breakfast.

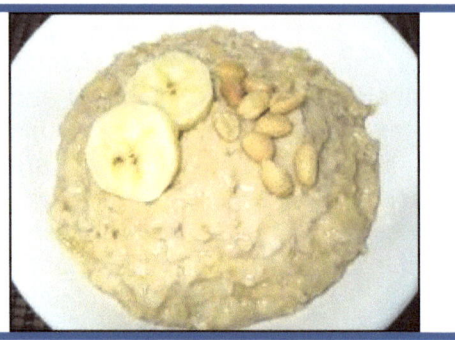

While efforts based upon diet may help to reduce LDL in some patients, they may not be enough in other patients. Another step would be to give the patient a drug that would either reduce LDL or increase HDL.

Statins are drugs that are widely used to reduce cholesterol. They reduce the synthesis of the critical enzyme on the pathway of cholesterol synthesis. And they also induce receptors for LDL in the liver, so that LDL in blood is taken into the liver. This reduces the amount of cholesterol in blood. Furthermore, as more LDL gets taken into the liver, the overall cholesterol inside the liver gets goes up. This reduces the amount of cholesterol made by liver.

The precursor in the pathway for making cholesterol is also used to make CoQ, a substance required in mitochondria. Since statins inhibit the production of the precursor of both cholesterol and CoQ, there is a danger that the CoQ levels will become too low. If this happens, muscle weakness will result, since muscles require the ATP's that are produced by mitochondria. The physician will monitor her patient for any muscle weakness, and recommend reducing the dosage of statins or perhaps using CoQ supplements, if needed.

Other drugs that increase the production of HDL are available. The physician may recommend a combination of drugs.

8.7. Summary

Lipoproteins in the blood transport fat and cholesterol. Chylomicrons transport fat and cholesterol from food in the diet. LDL (low density lipoprotein) transports fats made in the liver. HDL (high density lipoprotein) is the third major lipoprotein. High HDL and low LDL are associated with low risk of heart disease and stroke. The opposite is also true: low HDL and high LDL indicates an increased risk of hear disease and stroke.

9. Repair of the engine

9.1. All motors need repair

Sometimes you may lose a hubcap from your car. The battery may wear out. Or you may have a fender-bender. You can repair the car by buying a new hubcap or battery or by knocking out dents in the fender.

Materials from cells sometimes go astray or become damaged too. The theme of this chapter is how the cell replaces and salvages some materials and repairs others.

We are constantly being bombarded with dangerous substances, and even things that we need, can turn out to cause harm. We need O_2 and light to survive, for example. But both are also dangerous. Vitamin D is formed when light interacts with our skin, and so light is beneficial. But too much light causes damage to DNA. Since DNA ultimately determines what proteins are made, when DNA is damaged, the regulation of protein synthesis can be impaired. This can lead to skin cancer. The same is true for O_2. We need O_2 at all times but O_2 can also form reactive species that can destroy proteins and DNA.

Every time that we breathe, and every time we are in light, reactive compounds are formed. For the most part, these compounds do not kill cells, because cells have mechanisms that restore damaged and lost molecules.

The pentose phosphate shunt pathway is a player in protecting our cells. The pentose phosphate shunt is tied in to the making of fatty acids by providing. NADPH used in making fat (Chapter 8). Proteins are sometimes damaged, and the pentose phosphate shunt aids in recovery of damaged protein. It does this by making NADPH, which is used for repair. We will also mention the importance of anti-oxidants in the diet. These compounds are also used to restore damaged molecules.

9.2 Protein damage in red blood cells is repaired by the pentose phosphate shunt

The purpose of red blood cells is to transport oxygen, O_2, from the lungs to the tissue. Red blood cells do not consume O_2 as they have no mitochondria and O_2, is required for oxidative phosphorylation. Consequently, the concentration of O_2 is higher in red blood cells than in other tissues.

Nucleic acid molecules such as DNA and RNA and protein molecules are fragile. Chemical reactions can destroy them. There are many reactions that can cause tissue damage. One type of these reactions is caused by what is called "reactive oxygen species", ROS.

ROS are toxic products of oxygen. One is the familiar hydrogen peroxide (H_2O_2) used to bleach hair. It does this by chemically destroying the pigment in hair. There are also other ROS's. Many of these are free radical species. In a free radical species the rules of chemical bonding (for instance one rule is that O has two bonds and C has four bonds) no longer hold. Free radical species are very reactive and can wreck havoc on proteins. Fire is an example of a free radical chemical reaction. Left alone, fire will rage until all the fuel is consumed. It is not good to have many free radical species in the body.

Several of the 20 amino acids that make up proteins contain sulfur, and these amino acids are susceptible to damage by ROS. One of these is cysteine, 3 C amino acid like alanine. The structure of cysteine is:

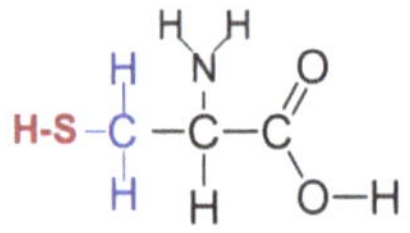

The symbol for sulfur is S. In proteins, the -SH group is called a sulfhydral group. SH groups in proteins are usually on the surface of the protein and exposed to the surrounding water.

The SH group is required for the proper function of many enzymes, but the –SH group is very reactive to ROS. When –SH reacts with ROS where the H from S is removed from -SH a free radical species forms.

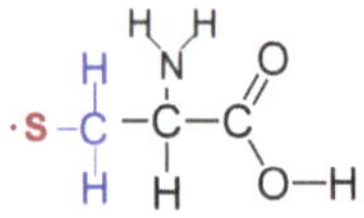

In the cell, two cysteine amino acids that are free radicals hook on to each other, forming a dimer (dimer means being composed of two single molecules or groups. The single molecule is called monomer). The dimer is called cystine and this is what it is:

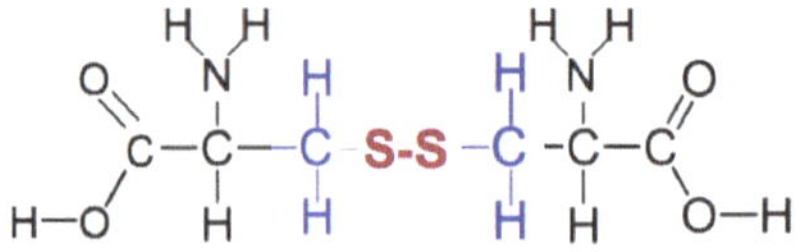

This reaction also occurs in proteins that contain cysteine. In the figure below, part of a peptide containing cysteine is shown. A whole peptide chain in a protein is much bigger than the peptide shown and the red blob illustrates the rest of the protein peptide chain.

Figure 9.1A This is a hypothetical protein that has two cysteine amino acids	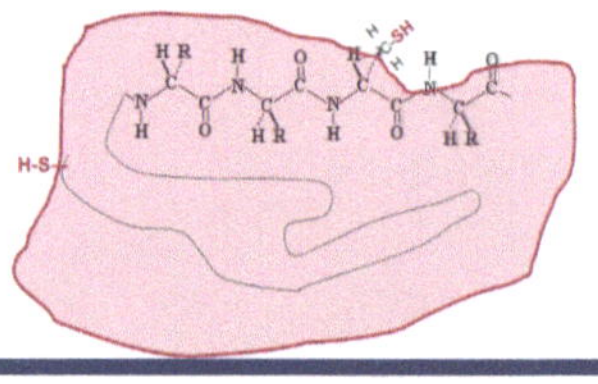
Figure 9.1B When the cysteine –SH group has an H removed, the free radical –S· is formed. Now two molecules can join. The two protein molecules are no longer attached to each other. They can form attachments with other protein molecules, and a big mess results.	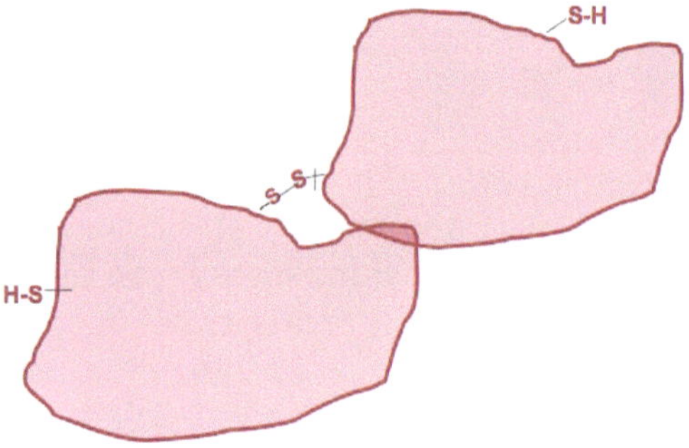

When proteins contain more than one cysteine, then the reactive free radical SH group can react with another. Cysteine, the SH form of the amino acid, is found in most proteins within cells. These proteins are functional only when the cysteine is in the SH form. In contrast, cystine, the dimeric form of cysteine that has –S-S-, is found in proteins found outside of cells. For instance, in the hormone insulin, an extracellular protein found in the blood plasma, the form is cystine.

9.3 How to keep proteins within cells in the SH form

The pentose-phosphate shunt pathway (introduced in 7.3.2) keeps the amino acid in the cysteine form for nearly all proteins that are within cells. Since we always need O_2, ROS are always present and, at all times, there must be a way to repair proteins with damaged SH groups.

One could imagine that the damaged protein could be repaired using a specialized "repair" enzyme. But there are many proteins in the cell, and each type of protein would need its own repair enzyme. Instead, a small compound called glutathione repairs all SH groups. Glutathione is composed of three amino acids that we have seen before: glutamic acid, cysteine and glycine. Figure 9.2 shows that glutathione attacks S-S bonds by adding H atoms. In so doing, it becomes a S free radical, which reacts with another S free radical to form glutathione disulfide.

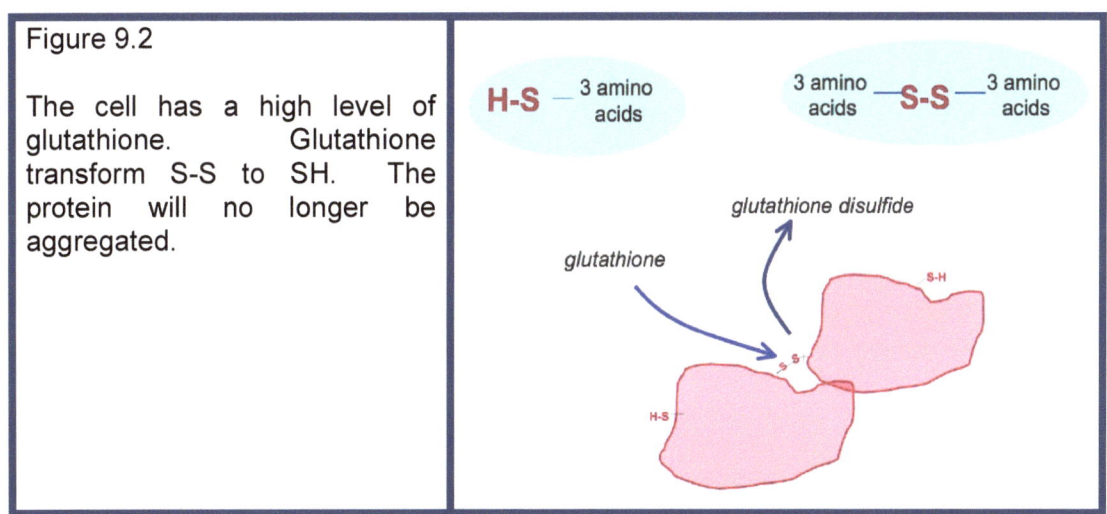

Figure 9.2

The cell has a high level of glutathione. Glutathione transform S-S to SH. The protein will no longer be aggregated.

This molecule repairs the free radical S groups, but in turn it gets transformed to a S-free radical molecule. Then NADPH, from the pentose phosphate shunt pathway, repairs glutathione, using just one enzyme, called glutathione reductase. Notice the "trick" that the cell uses. There are many reactive species reactive species made. To repair these many species, one compound, glutathione is used. Then a single enzyme system using NADPH restores the glutathione.

NADPH is formed in the cytoplasm by the pentose-phosphate shunt. The pentose-phosphate shunt is indicated in blue:

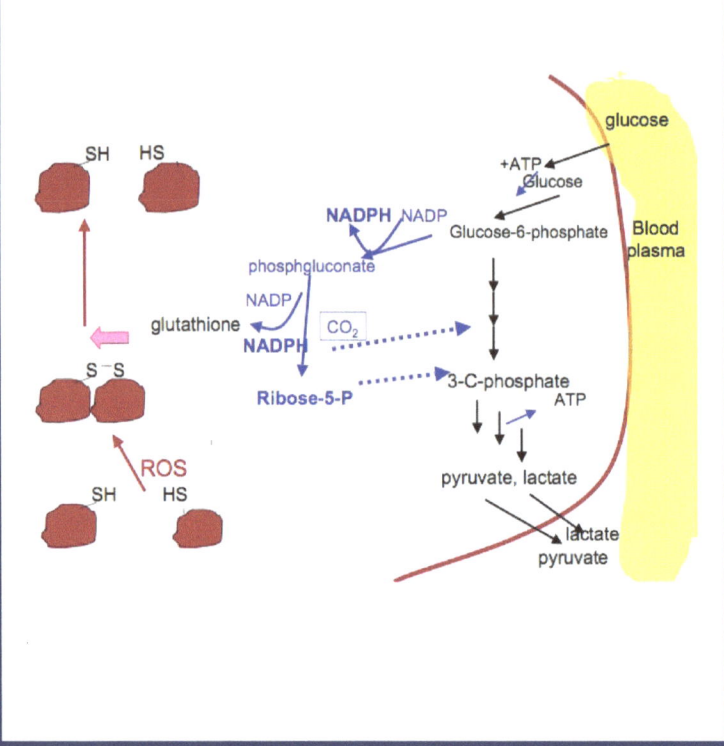

Figure 9.3

ROS stands for Reactive Oxygen Species. The black part of the figure shows glycolysis. The pentose-phosphate shunt is shown in blue.

ROS damages protein by causing cysteines to bind to other cysteine residues. This makes the proteins aggregate. Glutathione restores the cysteine. Glutathione itself forms a bond with another glutathione molecules in the process. NADPH restores the glutathione.

Glucose-6-phosphate is obtained glucose from the breakdown of glycogen or coming in from the blood. The products of glycolysis are pyruvate and lactate, which, for red blood cells go back into the blood and ultimately get metabolized by the liver. But not all of the glucose-6-phosphate goes to pyruvate. When NADP levels are high some glucose-6-phosphate reacts with NADP to form NADPH and ultimately ribose-5-P. The first enzyme in this pathway is called glucose-6-phosphate dehydrogenase. This enzyme is inhibited when NADPH is high. This means that the enzyme does not work, and most of the glucose-6-phosphate is metabolized through glycolysis. But when NADPH is transformed into NADP in the repair of S groups, then the enzyme is active. Glucose-6-phosphate is transformed into phosphogluconate and NADPH is formed.

9.4 Pentose phosphate shunt in disease

When proteins within the cell aggregate inappropriately, they no longer act in the way that they should. Disease occurs. The first case describes a disease that affects primarily the red blood cells. Hemoglobin is densely packed in RBC's. When the SH are damaged, hemoglobin molecules will bind to each other.

Case 1 (Milner et al., Blood 43, 271-276 (1974): A 39 year-old male, H. I., entered a hospital for an unrelated condition. It was observed that his skin and sclera (whites of eyes) had a yellow tinge. ILaboratory results are below:

	patient	control
Hemoglobin, g/dl	12	13-15
Reticulocyte count, %	25	0.5 - 2
Total bilirubin, mg/dl	3.9	0.2-1.2
Appearance of red blood cells	Heinz bodies	No Heinz bodies

The physicians were alerted to a possible problem for H. I. by the yellow color of his skin and sclera, and this suggests a problem called jaundice, which means bilirubin is high. Indeed, testing showed that bilirubin in his blood is high. Bilirubin is a break-down product of heme. Heme is the substance that binds O_2 in hemoglobin. Bilirubin can be high because too much is produced or not enough is removed. Some new-born babies have high bilirubin, leading to jaundice (also yellow skin and sclera). This can occur in premature babies because the liver is sometimes not developed enough to contain the enzymes that break-down bilirubin and lead to bilrubin excretion. For the baby, high bilirubin is due to under-consumption. The body produces the normal amount of bilirubin, but the level is high because it is not removed fast enough.

H.I. is not a new-born baby, but we can still ask whether there may be a problem with bilirubin removal. However, the observation of high reticulocytes is another clue. Reticulocytes are young red blood cells. They have a nucleus that can be seen under a microscope. As the cells mature, they lose the nucleus; mature red blood cells have no nucleus.

The observation of elevated reticulocytes is characteristic of a hemolytic anemia. This occurs because the red blood cells do not last for their usual 120 days, but are lysed, i.e., they break open. Therefore, the percentage of young cells in the blood increases. When red blood cells are reduced, a hormone called erythropoietin is produced that stimulates the production of new red blood cells. The high reticulocytes suggest that red blood cells are broken down but H.I. does not become severely anemic because the synthesis of new red blood cells compensates.

The red blood cells appeared abnormal under the microscope. They had dark enclosures. These features are called "Heinz bodies". They are aggregated hemoglobin molecules. (Think of dried up catsup around a catsup bottle, and you have a way to remember what Heinz bodies look like!)

Discussion, diagnosis and treatment of H.I.: Red blood cells of H.I. were studied. The researchers found that the enzyme glucose-6-phosphate dehydrogenase was defective in H.I. so production of NADPH was reduced. This resulted in the Heinz bodies in the RBC's, and led to fragility of the RBC's.

Glucose-6-phosphatase dehydrogenase (G6PD) deficiency is a common disease-producing enzymopathy (a disease produced by abnormal enzyme) in humans. One amino acid of G6PH in H.I has been changed to another one. H.I. has a mild form of the disease. Reactive ROS increase with severe infection, and with some drugs including antimalarial drugs. A substance in fava beans also produce ROS's. In these cases, the patient may have a hemolytic attack. The patient should be advised not to use certain drugs or eat fava beans. In case of a hemolytic attack he can be treated by dialysis and blood transfusion.

G6PD deficiency is inherited as an X-linked disorder and it affects 400 million people worldwide. There are many variants of G6PD deficiency and that one that H.I. has is called the Manchester variant, named after the English city where it was discovered. G6PD deficiency confers protection against malaria, which probably accounts for its high gene frequency. The variant is prevalent in people of Mediterranean origin. H.I. came from England, and the variant is not uncommon in the British Isles. (Remember, England was once a Roman colony).

> **Case 2: Cancer patient receiving radiation.** A 49 year-old female, J.K., was diagnosed with breast cancer, specifically ductal carcinoma. She was treated by surgery, followed by chemotherapy and then radiation. X-ray treatment occurred each day for 30 consecutive days. The radiologist suggested an arm exercise that exercises the pectoral muscle that was below the radiation site. What metabolic pathways would be in play with these exercises and how might that aid in repair of the muscle from the radiation damage?
>
> *Discussion:* X-ray beams break chemical bonds forming free radical species. Within a short time these species transform SH groups in proteins to S free radicals that can react with other S free radical species to make –S-S- bonds. Exercise increases Ca levels in the muscle, and stimulates glycogen breakdown to glucose-6-phosphate. Glucose-6-phosphate is the starting compound for the pentose-phosphate shunt. When NADPH is low the enzyme that transforms glucose-6-phosphate to phosphogluconate with the production of new NADPH is stimulated. Exercise, therefore, could help to help repair the free radicals and to lessen damage to protein. This explanation is an hypothesis only, however, since there is little experimental evidence to support this.

9.5 Other substances that are anti-oxidants

ROS produces free radicals when it reacts with fatty substances, DNA, RNA, proteins and other molecules. Vitamin C and vitamin E are two substances that are antioxidants. Vitamin C is involved in collagen formation. Collagen is a protein that is extracellular, and it is used for structure – it holds tissues together. Lack of vitamin C leads to the disease called scurvy, characterized by malaise, skin and gum disorders.

Vitamin E is not water soluble, and it is thought to protect the fatty acid part of membranes from oxidation. Neurological problems occur with vitamin E deficiency. β-carotene and polyphenol are other anti-oxidants that are soluble in the fatty acid part of membranes.

Clinical trials are mostly inconclusive for possible benefits of other anti-oxidant supplements. Just because something is an anti-oxidant in the test tube does not mean it will be anti-oxidant in the body. There must be enzymes in the body that will use the particular anti-oxidant molecule. But there are credible studies showing people who eat diets rich in fruits and vegetables, foods rich in antioxidants, have health benefits.

9.6 Salvaging adenosine

ATP is the dollar bill of metabolism. Just as money is needed to keep the economy going, the energy produced when ATP loses a phosphate to make ADP is required to keep metabolism going.

Here are the components of ATP:

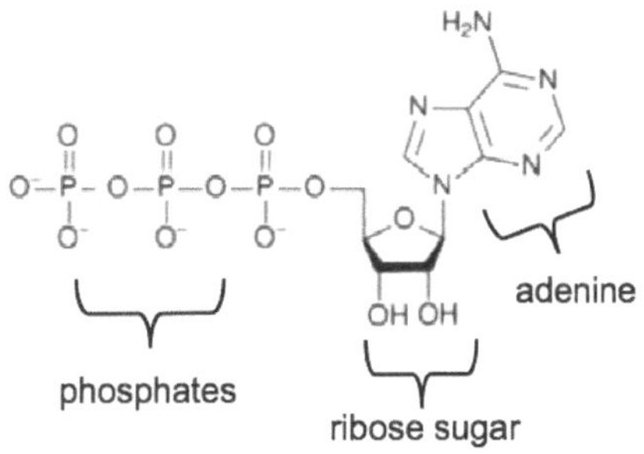

Our bodies make adenosine from basic small molecules, but it is "expensive" to do so. Many ATP reactions of ATP going to ADP are required to make adenosine.

Although, ADP gets phosphorylated to cycle back to ATP, there is a gradual decline in the amount of ADP and ATP in cells. We can understand this by looking at the reactions of ATP. When there is a demand for energy ATP goes to ADP with the release of P.

$$ATP \rightarrow ADP + P$$

In tissues where demand is suddenly high, there is a way to get ATP from ADP. The enzyme **myokinase** catalyzes this reaction:

$$2\ ADP \rightarrow ATP + AMP$$

This is an "emergency" reaction; it gives ATP when there is a sudden and large need for extra ATP to provide energy. Myokinase was first found in muscles (the preface "myo" means muscle) and but it is also found in other cells, including the nervous system.

AMP can be further degraded to for adenosine and the ribose sugar. The ribose sugar is metabolized to to 3 C units, as shown in Figure 1, and then ultimately to CO_2 in the citric acid cycle.

The adensoine part is also finally degraded. Oxygen atoms are attached to it, forming the compound urate. Urate is a waste product and it is excreted into the urine.

High levels of urate is associated with disease. When urate is too high in the blood, urate crystals can form. This can lead to renal stones and to the condition called gout, where crystals of urate form in joints, especially the joints of toes. This is a painful condition,[5]

---

[5] Many famous people have suffered from gout, including Thomas Jefferson, Henry VIII, John Calvin, Benjamin Disraeli, Karl Marx and Pope Clement VIII.

To save energy required to make more adenosine, and to reduce the amount of urate excreted in the urine, the body salvages the adenine. More than 90% of the AMP broken down does not get excreted from the body, but is salvaged.

The ability to reclaim adenosine and transform it back to AMP, and then ADP and ATP is found in all tissues. Here is the pathway for breakdown and salvage.

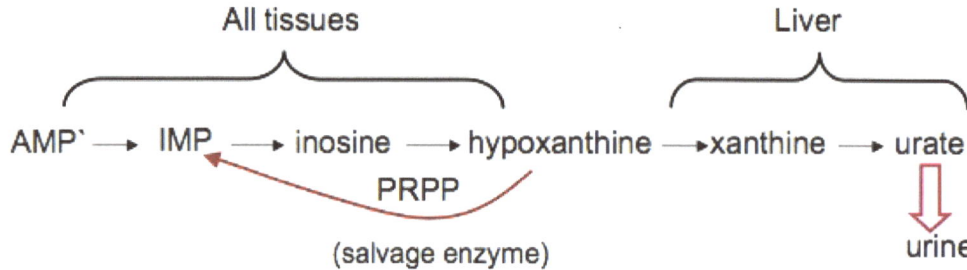

AMP gets transformed to IMP, and then the ribose sugar gets taken off. The product is inosine. Inosine gets transferred into hypoxanthine. Hypoxanthine can diffuse out of the cell into the blood. But most of the hypoxanthine gets the sugar put back on it to form IMP. The sugar is a 5 C sugar, pentose, made by the phosphopentose shunt. Once the sugar is added, IMP can be transformed into AMP. AMP is phosphorylated by myokinase (above) and oxidative phosphorylation to make ATP. The liver also has these salvage enzymes, but the liver can convert hypoxanthine to urate by adding oxygen atoms. Urate formed in the liver goes into the blood, and then is excreted in the urine.

9.7 Too much urate acid: gout and kidney stones

There are several general reasons why high urate in the blood might occur. One is that too much is produced. Too much produced may be due to altered enzymes in the synthesis. It can also be due to impaired salvage pathway.

The following case is a very rare disease, in which the salvage pathway is missing.

> **Case**: Patient, L.M. was a full term baby. At three months he was weak and cried excessively. He was late in sitting up and never learned to walk. At age three he began to bite his lips and fingers. He bit his fingers so much that he literally ate them and he lost the fingers on one hand. As he grew older he developed kidney stones and gout. He never learned to speak.

> **Diagnosis, treatment and discussion**: This describes a patient with Lesch-Nyhan syndrome, where the salvage enzyme is lacking. All of the hypoxanthine gets transformed into urate. The neurological problems are probably related to the lack of sufficient ATP in the nerve cells, but the bizarre behavior is not understood. A drug called allopurinal partially inhibits the enzyme that forms uric acid. In this case hypoxanthine increases in the blood. Hypoxanthine is excreted in the urine. The patient's blood will also have a mixture of hypoxanthine, xanthine and urate. A mixture also inhibits the formation of urate crystals. Allopurinal helped relieved L.M.'s gout, but did not reverse the severe

neurological problems.   No one understands why these patients have the neurological problems.

This disease is linked to the x chromosome, and so it is seen more in boys than in girls. Although this is a very rare disease, this disease illustrates the importance of salvaging adenosine, since without salvage the patient is very sick.

Another reason for high urate is under-secretion, i.e. the body does not properly get rid of urate. This is the more common reason, and is often seen in the elderly. As people age, the kidney function often decreases. The kidney does not remove the urate fast enough and urate levels increase.

Case: L.M. is a 74 year old male. He has had high glucose in his blood, and the doctor prescribed metformin for this. He has arthritis in the knees and for 10 years he has taken aspirin to control pain. In spite of this, he drinks a six-pack of beer every day and often has a shot of whiskey in the evening. In the last two weeks his left toe became red, swollen and painful. He cannot walk on it. It is even painful to have a blanket on the toe when he is sleeping.

Diagnosis, treatment and discussion: Blood tests showed high urate in the blood. L.M. is drinking mainly alcohol, not water. Urate levels became high because not enough water is going through his kidney. By drinking more water, more water goes through the kidney and this helps to dilute the urate. With age kidney function deteriorates; gout is often seen in the elderly because kidney function often deteriorates with age. Some medicines also have side effects of causing kidney malfunction. L.M. has high urate acid in his blood due to underexcretion of urate.

L.M. should be encouraged to drink more water and less alcohol. The physician should examine the patient for impaired kidney function. He should also look at the medicines the L.M. is taking to make sure that his meds do not contribute to kidney impairment.

10. Delivering oxygen

10.1 Oxygen is continually needed

We started the discussion of metabolism with this equation:

$$\text{Food} + O_2 \text{ (from air)} \rightarrow CO_2 + H_2O + \text{energy}$$

To obtain energy we need food and O_2. So far, we have been talking what happens to food -- C, H, O and N. The food part is explained through these basic concepts: foods are composed of fats, carbohydrates and protein, and the metabolism in each organ of the body depends upon its energy needs. But, as we study deeper, food metabolism becomes more complicated. Why is this? First of all, we eat so many things. Therefore, metabolism must be flexible. Second, we store fats, carbohydrates and proteins. Mechanisms are needed to both store fuel and retrieve it from storage when needed. Third, we do so many things. The mobilization of food from storage depends on activity, food intake and stress level and it depends upon the cooperation of all the organs of the body.

Unlike the metabolism of food, the other part of metabolism is easy. We use O_2 – and nothing else -- to convert the C's and H's in food to CO_2 and H_2O. O_2 is used in the mitochondria and it is essential for producing ATP. We do not store vast supplies of O_2, so we need to breathe air containing O_2 at all times.

The body uses interesting, intricate means to insure the delivery of O_2 to all tissues. Two protein molecules, involved in O_2 transport, are **myoglobin** and **hemoglobin**. Hemoglobin is in red blood cells (RBC's) and it makes blood red. O_2 binds to hemoglobin in the lungs and releases O_2 in capillaries. When O_2 is released in the capillary, O_2 molecules diffuse across the capillary wall and across the cell membrane, and go through the cell to the mitochondria where they are used. Aerobic muscle cells contain myoglobin. Myoglobin binds O_2 and gives a small extra amount of O_2 reserve for the muscle cells. Myoglobin is also red, and it gives aerobic muscles a red or brownish color.

Special properties of myoglobin and hemoglobin ensure that O_2 is delivered to tissue where it is needed. Myoglobin binds O_2 in a simple manner: the more O_2 around, the more O_2 is bound to myoglobin until all myoglobin molecules have O_2 bound to them. Hemoglobin, on the other hand, is more complicated. It binds O_2 tighter in the lung where O_2 is high, and less tightly in the tissue, where O_2 is low. Both taking in O_2 in the lung and release of O_2 in the tissue is achieved by this means. Two pathways, the glycolytic pathway and the citric acid cycle, indirectly play a role in assisting the binding and release of O_2 from hemoglobin.

10.2 First the big picture on how O_2 is transported to tissue

Oxygen, O_2, surrounds us in the atmosphere. Oxygen comprises 20% of the atmosphere. It is at the surface of every part of the body. We might think that we could use this oxygen – that we would not need to breathe. But, O_2 is not very soluble in water and we are made up of mostly water. Only very little O_2 diffuses through the skin. Lungs, heart, blood vessels and blood are all needed to deliver O_2 to tissue.

| Figure 10.1. Picture of capillary and two cells that do not contain myoglobin.

Red blood cells (RBC) are red, and contain hemoglobin. Blood plasma is indicated by yellow, and plasma contains glucose, amino acids, fatty acids, lipoproteins. O_2 is released from hemoglobin, and O_2 diffuses through the capillary wall into the cell, and into the mitochondria. | 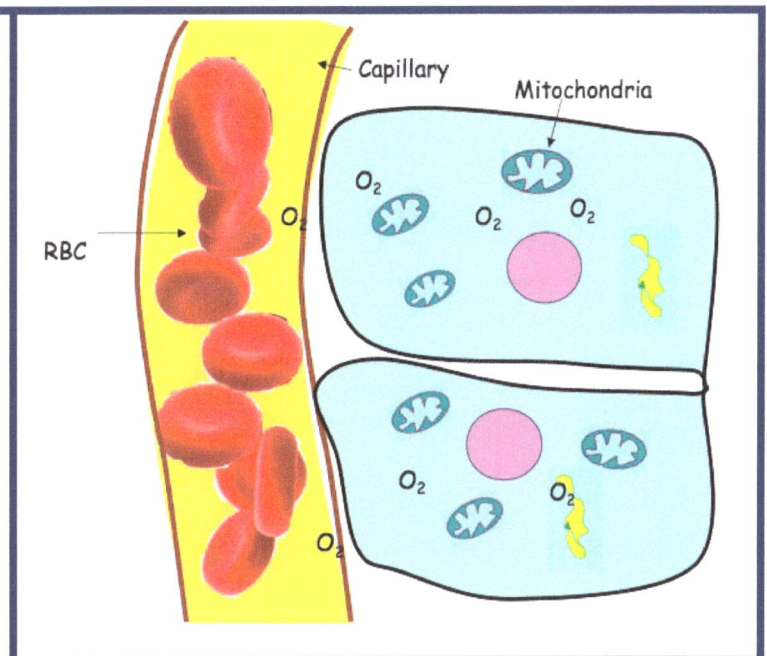 |

When GB is skateboarding or mountain climbing, GB's muscles need more ATP and to make ATP in the mitochondria O_2 is needed. There is a sensor for O_2 in the carotid artery. When O_2 in the blood gets low and CO_2 produced from metabolism gets high, a signal gets sent from chemical sensors in the carotid artery and aorta to the area of the brain that controls breathing rate. GB begins to breathe faster and the heart beats faster. More O_2 is delivered to the tissue as the blood circulates through the body faster. This is a short-term, immediate response to the acute need for O_2.

Long term response of the body also occurs when O_2 in the blood is low. Specialized cells in the kidney sense low O_2 and excrete the hormone erythropoietin. Erythropoietin stimulates the production of red blood cells (RBC's) in the bone marrow. More RBC's are made. After a person loses blood, blood RBC's and hemoglobin will be restored by the stimulus of erythropoietin. When RBC's are initially made they have a nucleus. RBC's with a nucleus are called reticulocytes. Within a few days of circulating in the blood, they lose the nucleus. Since nuclei have DNA, which has the information for protein synthesis, mature RBC's without a nucleus cannot make protein. As they get older, the cells suffer damage and finally after about 120 days the spleen removes old RBC's. In normal blood, about 1 – 2 % of RBC's are reticulocytes, the new RBC's with a nucleus.

Under conditions of chronic, long-term O_2 deprivation, more capillaries form. This can happen when living for a long time at high altitudes and some people living at high altitude in the Andes have this condition. Formation of more capillaries may also occur in people who are suffering from a weakened heart. The complexion of these patients may appear red due to more capillaries in their tissue.

Breathing faster, increasing blood circulation and making more hemoglobin along with more RBC's are some ways that O_2 delivery to tissue is regulated. But the molecules myoglobin and hemoglobin, both of which carry O_2, need to be examined to understand how O_2 is delivered.

10.3 Myoglobin in muscle cells

Myoglobin binds O_2 in red muscle, which are dependent upon mitochondria to give ATP. Myoglobin serves as a small store of O_2 in this tissue and gives red meat its color. Figure 2 shows a picture of the capillary, and a mitochondrial-rich red muscle cell. The inset is a picture of myoglobin.

Figure 10.2.	
Picture of a capillary and muscle cell that contains myoglobin. Red muscle cells contain myoglobin. The blow-up shows a picture of myoglobin. Green shows the part that is made up of amino acids. An iron atom resides within a heme group where the arrow is pointing. Oxygen binds to iron. The symbol for iron is Fe.	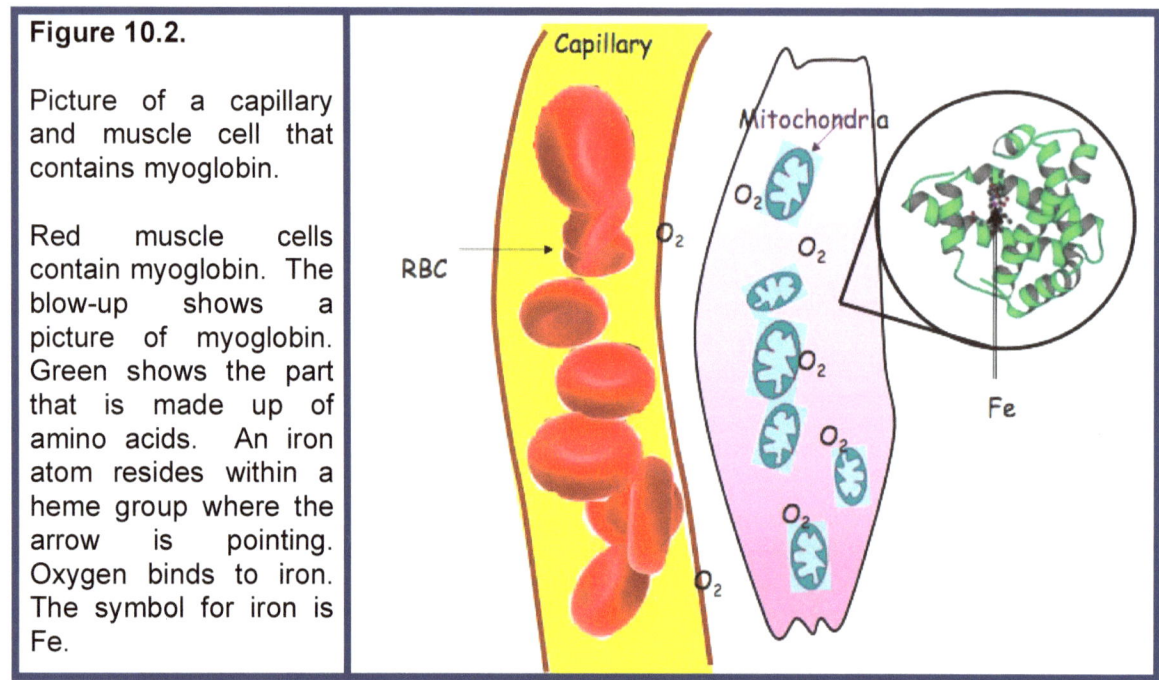

Iron (Fe) is in the center of myoglobin. O_2 binds to the iron atom. When O_2 concentration is high, more myoglobin will bind O_2. For those of you who like equations[1], here is the equation that describes this:

$$\frac{[\text{myoglobin with bound } O_2]}{[\text{Total myoglobin}]} = \frac{[O_2]}{K_m + [O_2]}$$

This equation is explained as follows. First, everything inside brackets [ ] refers to concentration. So $[O_2]$ says how much O_2 there is in a given volume. (Chemists usually use the units of moles in a liter. But you can say pounds in a quart too). When there is no O_2, then $[O_2]$ equals zero and there will be no O_2 bound to myoglobin. Therefore, the value of the left side of the equation is zero too. K_m is a constant that tells you the concentration when half of the myoglobin has O_2 bound to it. You can see that when $[O_2]$ equals K_m, the value of the right hand side of the equation is 0.5. When O_2 levels are very

---

[1] This equation is also for those of you who will study Biochemistry further. The same equation describes enzyme kinetics, i.e. how the speed of an enzyme-catalyzed reaction depends upon the substance being acted upon). If you continue in studying medicine, you will see this equation and binding curve many times! In pharmacology, this equation is called the "dose response curve." It says that at low dosage, giving higher amounts of drug produces a response. The amount of drug for 50% response is the K_m. At a high dosage giving more drug gets no more response.

high, then the left hand part of the equation is 1, telling you that all myoglobin molecules have O_2 bound to them.

Here is what the binding of O_2 to myoglobin looks like:

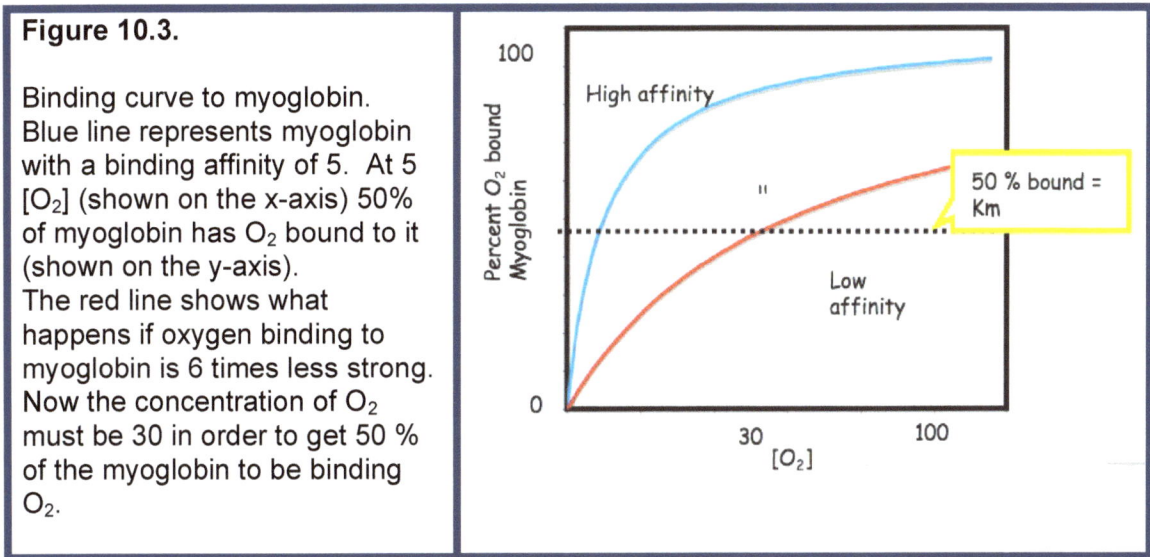

Figure 10.3.

Binding curve to myoglobin. Blue line represents myoglobin with a binding affinity of 5. At 5 $[O_2]$ (shown on the x-axis) 50% of myoglobin has O_2 bound to it (shown on the y-axis).
The red line shows what happens if oxygen binding to myoglobin is 6 times less strong. Now the concentration of O_2 must be 30 in order to get 50 % of the myoglobin to be binding O_2.

The curve in Figure 10.3 shows that as O_2 concentration increases, more and more O_2 gets bound to myoglobin until all the myoglobin has O_2 bound to it. Looking back at the equation when O_2 goes very high, the right hand side of the equation comes close to 1, and then the left hand part of the equation is 1, i.e., 100% of myoglobin has O_2 bound to it. The dotted line in the graph shows the point where 50% of the myoglobin has O_2 bound to it. K_m is a constant that tells you the concentration of O_2 when myoglobin has 50% of the molecules with O_2 bound. When you look at the equation, you will see that when O_2 equals K_m then the value of the left hand side is 0.5, meaning that 50 % of myoglobin has O_2 bound. When myoglobin does not bind very well, the K_m value will be higher -- it takes more O_2 to get 50% bound.

The equation describes a general binding curve. Let us consider the red muscle cells again. When O_2 is high most of the myoglobin has bound O_2. When muscle contracts O_2 is consumed in the mitochondria to make ATP. Suddenly the O_2 concentration is lower. Then some of the the O_2 from myoglobin is released, giving the cells an extra bit of O_2. In this way, myoglobin acts as a small store of O_2.

10.4 Oxygen binding to hemoglobin

RBC's, containing many hemoglobin molecules, are cells that are circulating in blood. Hemoglobin molecules within the cells need to pick up O_2 in the lungs and release it in the capillaries.

But, for this simple function, hemoglobin has very interesting properties that differ from myoglobin. Although, hemoglobin resembles myoglobin, hemoglobin is four times bigger and it has four protein peptide chains. Each peptide chain has an iron atom in it and each iron atom can bind one O_2 molecule. The inset in Figure 10.4 shows what a hemoglobin molecule looks like.

Figure 10.4.	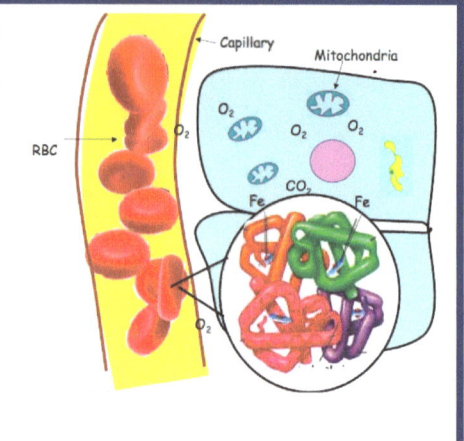
Hemoglobin has 4 protein or polypeptide chains, shown in different colors. There are two pairs of polypeptide chains; one is called alpha chain and the other is beta chain. Hemoglobin has 4 Fe (iron) atoms; each polypeptide has one Fe atom. Each polypeptide chain in hemoglobin is similar to one myoglobin molecule. Myoglobin can bind one O_2 molecule. Hemoglobin can bind four O_2 molecules.	

With little O_2 around, the protein does not bind O_2 with high affinity. The protein is called "T" for taut or tight. The polypeptide chain wraps tightly around the iron making it hard for O_2 to bind. Therefore, you need a high concentration of O_2 for binding. Conversely, bound O_2 does not stay bound to hemoglobin. What is bound to hemoglobin, gets released to the tissues. By this means, the tissues, which are low in O_2 gets O_2 delivered to them.

After one or two O_2 molecule is bound to one or two irons, the protein changes. The polypeptide chain now wraps around looser around the iron. It wraps in a "relaxed" manner, making it easier for O_2 to bind. The protein conformation is now called "R" for relaxed. The result of this change is that the initial binding of O_2 makes it easier for hemoglobin to bind more O_2. This is what happens in the lung. The hemoglobin molecule "likes" to have when there are many O2 molecules around. Therefore, in the lungs, it binds O_2.

The diagram on Figure 5 shows how initial binding of O_2 to hemoglobin makes more O_2 bind with stronger affinity:

Figure 10.5	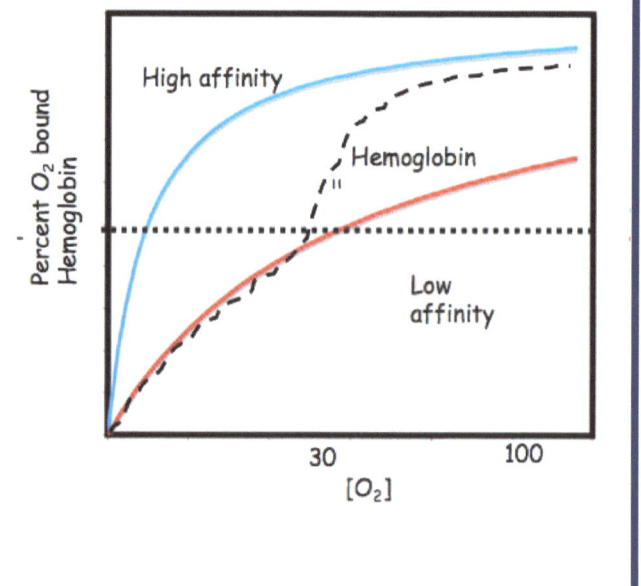
At low O_2 concentrations, hemoglobin binds O_2 with low affinity. At high O_2 concentrations, hemoglobin binds O_2 tightly, high affinity. The final result is that the binding of O_2 to hemoglobin is "cooperative". Hemoglobin binds O_2 tightly at high concentrations. Hemoglobin switches between a protein that binds O_2 loosely into one that binds O_2 tightly.	

Without hemoglobin's ability to change its ability to bind O_2, we would not survive. In the lungs where O_2 concentration is high, hemoglobin binds O_2 tightly. All or nearly all of the Fe molecules have O_2 bound to them. In the tissue, O_2 levels are low because mitochondria are using O_2. Then hemoglobin no longer binds O_2 tightly. It then releases the O_2 to the tissue.

The binding of O_2 to hemoglobin is said to be cooperative. When first molecule of O_2 binds it "cooperates" with the next O_2 molecule making it easier for the next one to bind. The transition from low affinity to high affinity binding is smoother than shown in Figure 10.5. Figure 10.6 shows the way O_2 binding to hemoglobin actually occurs when O_2 concentration is changed.

Figure 10.6	
This is what the cooperative binding of O_2 to hemoglobin looks like.	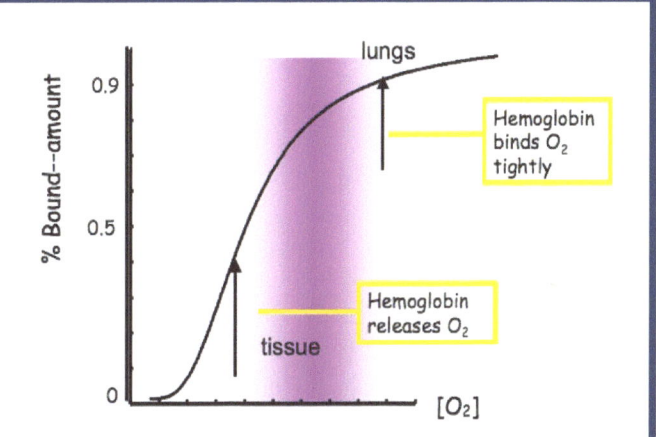
Hemoglobin binds O_2 tightly in the lungs where $[O_2]$ is high.	
In the tissue, $[O_2]$ is low and hemoglobin releases O_2 that is bound.	

Hemoglobin is a wonderful molecule. It is designed to pick up O_2 in the lungs where it binds O_2 tightly. Then it releases O_2 in the tissue, where O_2 concentration is low. This means that mitochondria in all of tissue in the body are supplied with O_2.

10.5 Metabolism affects O_2 release from hemoglobin

The interesting hemoglobin molecule has even more tricks. Metabolism has a direct effect on O_2 release. The goal is get as much O_2 from hemoglobin to the tissue as fast as possible.

The release of O_2 from hemoglobin occurs more readily at low pH. This statement causes several questions: What is pH? When and where is pH low in the blood? What produces the change in pH?

pH is a measure of H^+ ions. Water molecules, H_2O, separate to a small amount into H^+ and OH^- ions. The amount of H^+ and OH^- is small compared with the molecules of water present. H_2O is 55 M.[2] In neutral water, the concentration of H^+ is 0.0000001 M and OH-

---

[2] M is a symbol standing for the number of molecules in one liter. M stands for 630,000,000,000,000,000,000,000 molecules. Instead of writing that big number all the time, the symbol M is used. The normal glucose level in blood is 0.005 M. So the number of molecules in a liter of blood is 0.005 times that big number. Pure water is 55 M in H_2O. The number of water molecules in a liter of water is 55 times that big number.

is 0.0000001 M. The pH is 7 – indicating the number of zero's after the decimal point. When H^+ is bigger than OH^-, then a substance is considered acidic. For instance, the stomach fluid is acidic; its H^+ concentration is about 0.1 M after eating. This is equivalent to a pH of 1 – only one zero after the decimal point. Lemonade is also acidic. The pH of lemonade is about 4, indicating the H concentration is 0.0001 M.

For biological fluids, the number 7 is important to know. If the number gets lower, the fluid is acidic (more H than OH). If it is higher, it is basic (more OH than H). Normal pH of blood is about 7.3. When pH goes much lower than this (meaning that H^+ goes high) coma results. The brain does not work properly.

What changes the pH of blood in normal conditions?

It turns out that CO_2 does. CO_2 in water forms an acid. This is what happens when CO_2 is in water:

$$CO_2 + H_2O \rightarrow H_2CO_3 \rightarrow H^+ + HCO_3^-$$

CO_2 dissolves in water and forms H^+. This is how soda pop is made; CO_2 is put into water. The water becomes acidic and has a sharp -- and refreshing -- taste. Bubbles form as the CO_2 gradually goes out of the water.

We know where in the body CO_2 is formed. It is formed by the citric acid cycle and pyruvate dehydrogenase in mitochondria. When CO_2 is formed, it diffuses out of the cell into the capillaries. There it dissolves into the blood plasma and forms H^+ and HCO_3^-. Blood in the capillaries become more acidic. When hemoglobin is in an acidic environment, it binds O_2 less strongly. Therefore, the metabolite CO_2 aids in making hemoglobin release O_2 near the cells producing CO_2.

In the lungs CO_2 is exhaled. Then the reverse of the reaction occurs.

$$H^+ + HCO_3^- \rightarrow H_2CO_3 \rightarrow CO_2 + H_2O$$

Now when the lungs exhale CO_2, the pH goes up. At higher pH, hemoglobin binds O_2 tighter, and therefore more O_2 gets bound to hemoglobin in the lung.

There is another means to aid the release of O_2. As we stated, hemoglobin is in RBC's. The glycolysis pathway of RBC's produces ATP to maintain salt gradients. Glycolysis of RBC's has another function. One of the intermediates of glycolysis gets converted into a chemical called 2,3 BPG (bis-phosphoglycerate). This substance binds to hemoglobin and acts to make it more likely to release O_2 in the tissue.

Figure 10.7 shows the net result of these metabolic effects on hemoglobin binding.

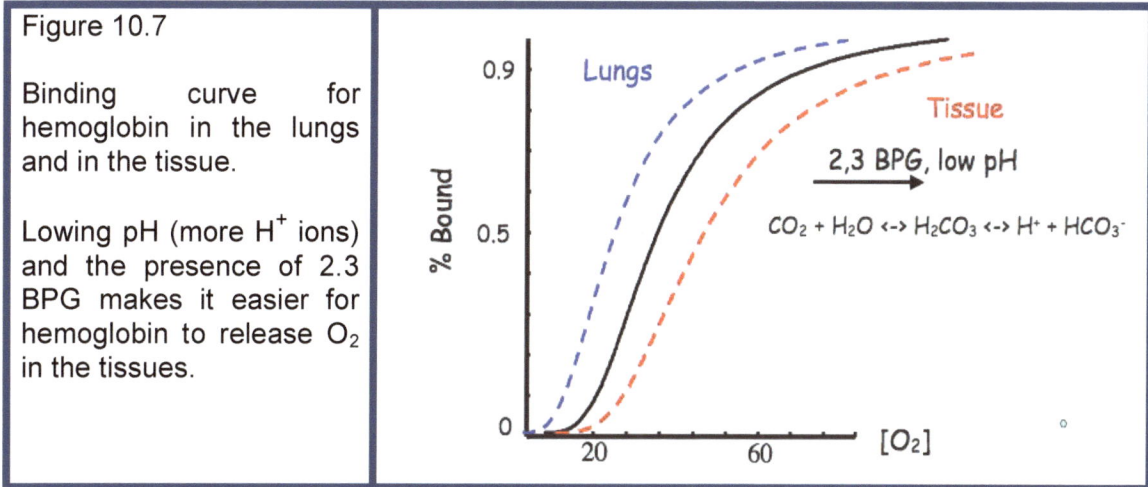

Figure 10.7

Binding curve for hemoglobin in the lungs and in the tissue.

Lowing pH (more H$^+$ ions) and the presence of 2.3 BPG makes it easier for hemoglobin to release O$_2$ in the tissues.

In the lungs, the high pH means hemoglobin binds O$_2$ tightly, with high affinity. In the tissue, the presence of 2,3 BPG and low pH means that O$_2$ binds to hemoglobin less tightly, and O$_2$ is released from hemoglobin.

So, the release of O$_2$ is influenced by metabolism of glucose in glycolysis, which makes 2,3 BPG. It is also influenced by the citric acid cycle in the mitochondria, which makes CO$_2$.

10.6 Cases involving anemia

Anemia is the word that describes the condition when RBC's and hemoglobin are low in the blood. When hemoglobin is low, O$_2$ delivery to tissues will be less. When a patient has low hemoglobin, the question is why. Whenever something is low, there are two possibilities: Not enough is being made, or it is being removed too fast.

Case 1. **Anemia in an adult woman**
ST is a 30 year old woman. In the past three years she has had three children. A son was born 3 years ago, and 6 months ago she delivered twins. The pregnancies and delivery were normal. She complains of fatigue.

Signs

	Patient	Normal
Blood hemoglobin	9.1 g/dl	12 to 14 g/dl
reticulocytes	1.5%	1 to 2
bilirubin	low	low

Discussion and treatment. The patient has low blood hemoglobin is severely anemic. Hemoglobin contains iron. When diet is insufficient in iron, the intestine does not absorb enough iron from food. If the patient loses iron by blood loss, the patient becomes iron deficient. Without iron, the body is no longer able to make enough hemoglobin. When hemoglobin levels go to 8 g/dl or below, the physician usually recommends a blood transfusion.

Iron deficiency is a common form of anemia, especially among women of child-bearing age. Blood loss occurs during menstruation and through pregnancies. Iron deficiency is an example of the case when not enough is being made.

111

Iron supplements are recommended, and the patient is counseled to eat iron rich foods. In iron deficiency hemoglobin is low because not enough is made, because iron is needed for the synthesis of hemoglobin.

Case 2: Anemia in a child.
Symptoms: Patient, A.B., is 8 year old boy was found to be tired and unable to keep up in playing with other children.   The whites of his eyes are yellow. (Yellowing is called icterus. Another name for this is jaundice).

Signs:

	Patient	Normal
Blood hemoglobin	10.1 g/dl	13 to 16 g/dl
reticulocytes	7 %	1 to 2
bilirubin	high	low

Diagnosis and treatment: This patient is suffering from hemolytic anemia. The word "lytic" means to break, and hemolytic anemia means that the RBC's are breaking down.
A clue for hemolytic anemia is the high level of reticulocytes. Reticulocytes are being formed, but the mature RBC's are not lasting as long as is normal. Consequently, the percentage of reticulocytes in the blood is high. The other clue for this is elevated bilirubin. Bilirubin is a break-down product of hemoglobin and it is metabolized by the liver and then excreted. Bilirubin gives a yellow color to the whites of eyes and a yellow tinge to the skin, and the patient is said to have jaundice.[3] For the patient here, the reason for bilirubin is "overproduction." Too much is being produced. The clue for this is the high reticulocytes which are being made in response to the break-down of RBC's.

With further enzyme tests, the physicians could determine that this patient has a defective pyruvate kinase, an enzyme of glycolysis. Pyruvate kinase is the last enzyme of glycolysis; it takes the phosphate on phosphoenolpyruvate, a 3 C intermediate of glycolysis to form ATP and pyruvate. Without enough ATP, the salt levels in the RBC's cannot be maintained, and the RBC's swell and are taken from circulation by the spleen. This is a genetic disease; it is a recessive disease, and so he inherited it from both his parents. There is a mutation in the portion of his DNA that makes pyruvate kinase.

A permanent cure for this patient would be gene therapy, whereby his DNA would be altered. However, although there is much work in this area, right now it is not possible to do this. The simple treatment is to give a blood transfusion when the hemoglobin becomes dangerously low. The disease is usually most noticeable in children during a growth spurt.

10.7 Anemia due to hemoglobin variants and relationship to malaria

Hemoglobin shows many variants, this is to say that people coming from different parts of the world often show slightly different kinds of hemoglobin. Many of these variants occur

---

3 Jaundice, due to high bilirubin, is sometimes seen in premature babies. The reason that these babies have high bilirubin is that their livers are not developed enough to remove the bilirubin.

in malaria-infected areas. Mosquitoes transmit the organism of Plasmodium to humans where it infects red blood cells as part of its life-cycle. During history most tropical and temperate parts of the world had malaria, and at present, 225 million people contract malaria in a year, as estimated by the World Health Organization.

Peoples living in malarial areas (now wet areas of the tropics and subtropics) have developed some resistance to malaria. In the past chapter, we mentioned a variant in the enzyme glucose-6-phosphate dehydrogenase. This variant enzyme is found in populations living near the Mediterranean, and it is thought to help in by making red blood cells fragile. When RBC's are infected with the parasite, a strain is put on the RBC's. Fragile RBC's lyse, i.e. break open, and the parasite is destroyed. Therefore, fragility in RBC's gives an advantage in resistance to malaria.

Variants of hemoglobin also give resistance to malaria. Hemoglobin molecules are very densely packed in the red blood cell – so dense that the hemoglobin molecules are nearly touching. One variant of hemoglobin is called sickle cell hemoglobin. In this disease, one amino acid on one chain of the hemoglobin is altered. This makes the hemoglobin molecule "sticky" and it binds to another hemoglobin molecule and so on, finally making a big fiber of hemoglobin molecules. This fiber distorts the RBC's. It is not so easy for distorted RBC's to go through capillaries. The RBC's tend to lyse and the life cycle of the parasite is interrupted. The sickle cell trait is common in sub-Saharan Africa.

Another variant of hemoglobin occurs when the chains of hemoglobin are not in the usual ratio. In most people hemoglobin is composed of two alpha chains and two beta chains. When more alpha chains are made than beta chains – or vice versa – a condition called thalessemia results. Hemoglobin with an unusual ratio of alpha to beta chains is less stable than hemoglobin with the usual 1:1 ratio. One type of thalessemia is found in people with origins in Southeast Asia and another type is found in people from the Mediterranean region.

Glucose-6-phosphate dehydrogenase deficiency, sickle cell hemoglobin and thalessemia diseases are inherited. A gene is inherited from both the father and mother. When a person is heterozygous, meaning that only one gene for the particular condition is present, the anemia is mild or even not noticeable. When the person is homozygous, meaning that the gene has been inherited from both father and mother, the anemia's are more pronounced.

11. Engine trouble: Diabetes and the homeostasis of glucose

11.1 Diabetes

One theme of this book on energy production has been the requirement of the brain to be supplied with glucose. The level of glucose in blood plasma is under tight homeostasis. The word homeostasis means that the level of glucose is regulated so that its level is approximately constant. When glucose gets high, the hormone insulin stimulates the pathways that remove glucose from the blood and converts glucose to storage forms of energy, namely glycogen and fat. When glucose is low, the hormones glucogon, epinephrine and cortisol stimulate the production of glucose so that the glucose blood level is stable. The production of keto-acids is stimulated during long-term starvation.

Diabetes is a disease where the regulation of sugar level in the blood is impaired. The manifestations of diabetes involve all the metabolic pathways. The National Institutes of Health estimates that diabetes affects 25.8 million people in the U.S. population. Nearly everyone in the U.S. either has the disease or has a friend or relative with the disease. Diabetes is a disease affecting the whole world. Research published in The Lancet estimated that 350 million people worldwide have diabetes, and that global diabetes rates doubled from 1980 to 2008.

Diabetes has various classifications. In Type I, or juvenile diabetes, pancreatic beta cells are destroyed, most likely by an infection or by an autoimmune response. They can no longer secrete enough insulin. In Type II diabetes the cells that have receptors to insulin become less sensitive to insulin. The beta cells respond by secreting more insulin, but ultimately they are overwhelmed.

By considering what happens when insulin is not present, we can review what we learned about metabolism.

11.2 Bringing glucose levels down: GB after feasting

We are going back to our patient, GB. Again GB eats a big piece of cake, and this time GB eats ice cream too. The sugar in his blood goes up. In response to high glucose levels, the pancreas secretes insulin. The ice cream supplies GB with protein too. High amino acids in the blood obtained from the protein meal also stimulate the release of insulin. Figure 11.1 shows the hormone response.

114

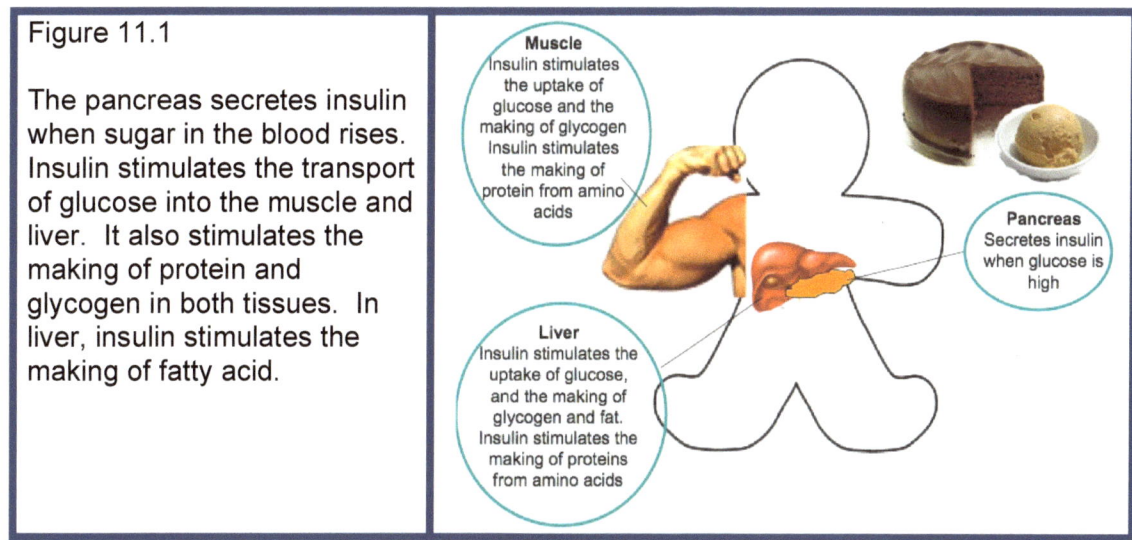

Figure 11.1

The pancreas secretes insulin when sugar in the blood rises. Insulin stimulates the transport of glucose into the muscle and liver. It also stimulates the making of protein and glycogen in both tissues. In liver, insulin stimulates the making of fatty acid.

Insulin stimulates all the pathways which remove glucose from the blood and which stores the C's supplied by carbohydrates and proteins. The general picture of insulin response in Figure 11.2 indicates that glycogen synthesis is enhanced, proteins are made in the muscles and other cells, fat is made in the liver, and fat is transported to the other tissues, especially to the adipose tissue.

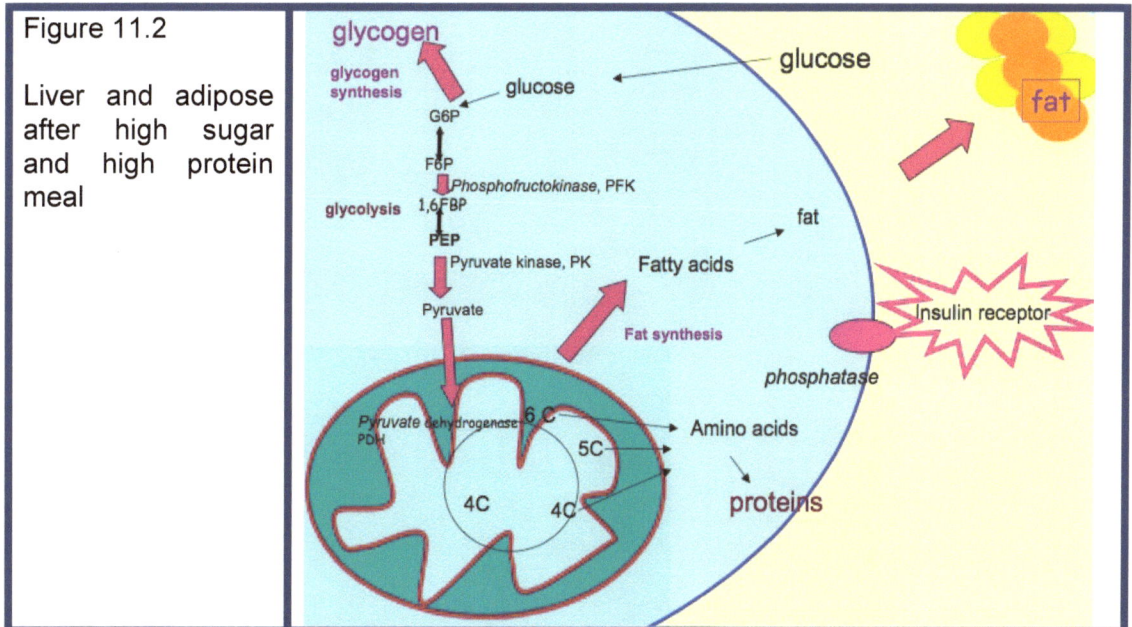

Figure 11.2

Liver and adipose after high sugar and high protein meal

11.3 Blood glucose levels of GB when fasting

Now we look at what happens when GB is not eating. Because the fuel comes from different sources and the source of fuel depends upon length of fasting and the energy requirements, a single hormone is not sufficient to release stored food. Three hormones are important during this nutritional period: glucogon, cortisol and adrenaline. Figure 11.3 shows the location where the three hormones are made. The three hormones stimulate the release of energy stores. Fuel comes from stored glycogen and fat and from protein.

| Figure 11.3.

Three hormones, glucogon, adrenalin and cortisone control the release of energy stores. | 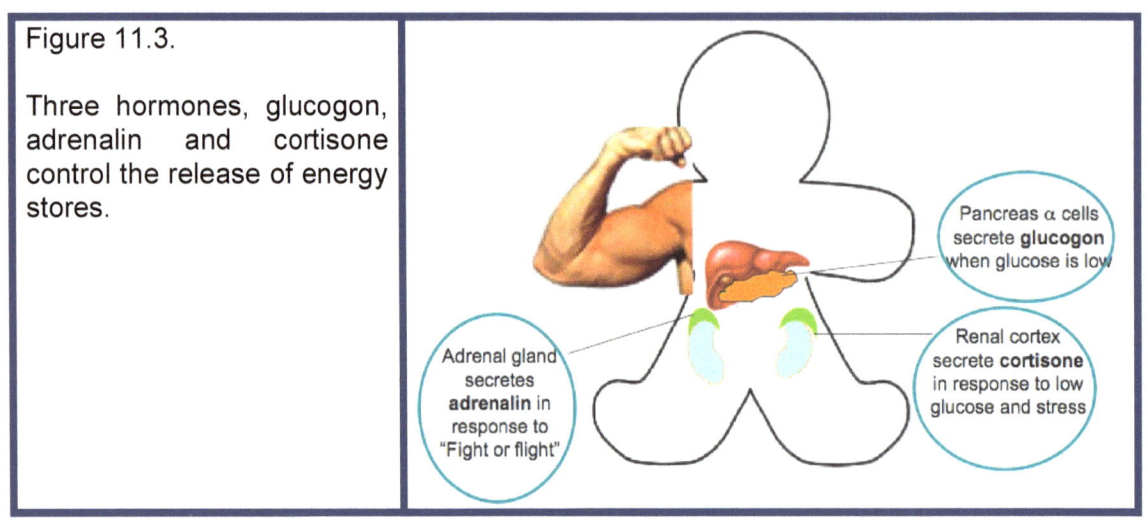 |

Figure 11.4 shows the pathways that are stimulated by adrenalin, glucogon and cortisol. These are the pathways that mobilize stored forms of food. Glycogen and fat are removed from tissue, and protein is broken down to form glucose.

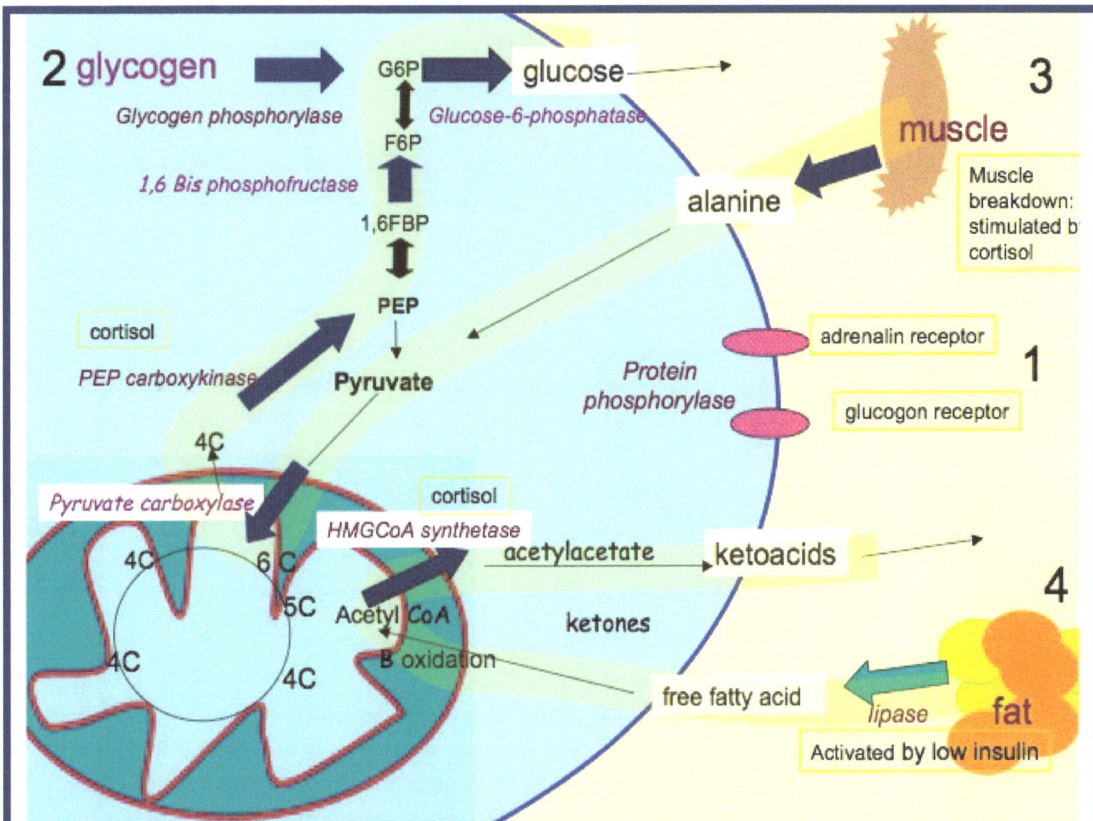

Figure 11.4. Mobilizing fuel during starvation conditions
The liver cell is shown in blue; blood plasma is yellow.

1. Receptors on the liver membrane bind adrenaline and glucogon. These receptors induce an enzyme called protein phosphorylase. This enzyme puts a phosphate on key enzymes that serve to mobilize fuel stores.

2. Glucogon stimulates enzymes that phosphorylate the enzymes that break down glygocen to form glucose-6-phosphate. This hormone plays a role in maintaining glucose levels during an overnight fast. The last step is breaking glucose-6-phosphate to glucose by the enzyme glucose-6-phosphase. This enzyme is only found in the liver.

3. Protein from muscle is broken down, in stimulation from cortisol. The major amino acid produced is alanine. Alanine gets converted into pyruvate in the liver; pyruvate is converted to glucose-6-phosphate by gluconeogenesis. The last step is breaking glucose-6-phosphate to glucose by the enzyme glucose-6-phosphase

4. Low insulin stimulates the lipase in fat cells. The lipase transforms triglyceride to free fatty acids. The free fatty acid gets transformed into acetyl CoA. The synthesis of enzyme HMGCoA synthetase is induced by cortisol. HMGCoA synthetase catalyzes the synthesis of acetoacetate, a ketoacid. This enzyme is found in the liver.

Now, GB does not eat for a long time, say, several days. Yet GB is healthy and alert. Under these conditions fatty acids are being used to make ketoacids. The transporters in the brain are altered and the brain uses ketoacids for fuel. Muscle also can use ketoacids for fuel. Muscles are broken down less rapidly than during beginning starvation; since ketoacids are used instead of glucose, there is less need for alanine to make glucose. Starvation is shown on Figure 11.5.

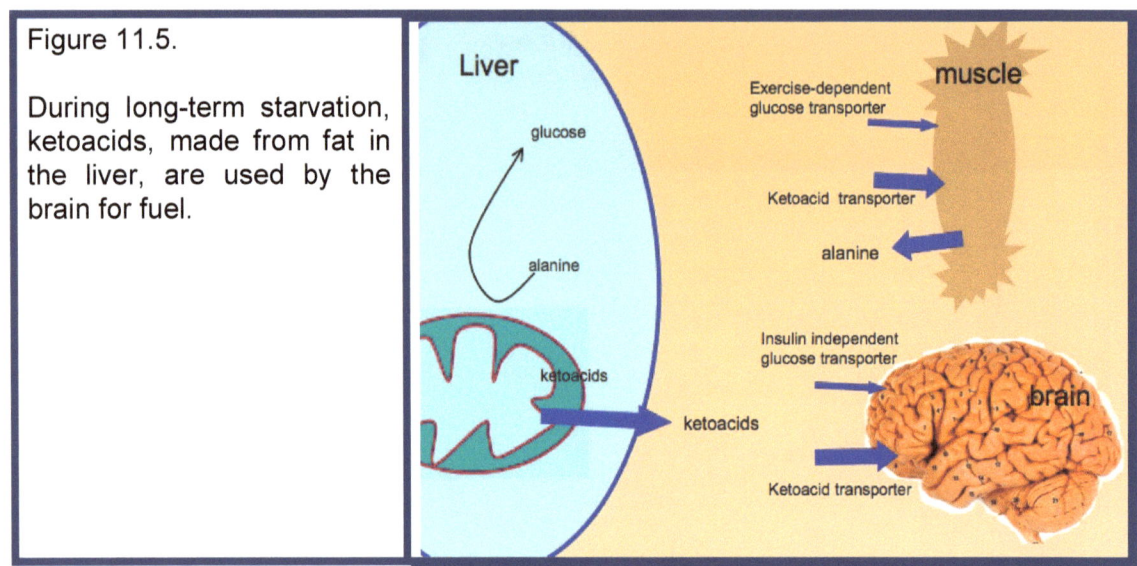

Figure 11.5.

During long-term starvation, ketoacids, made from fat in the liver, are used by the brain for fuel.

11.4 Case: what happens when a patient does not have insulin

Case: Coma in a student. A 20 year-old college student, XY, is admitted into the emergency room at 2:00 AM in a coma. He attended a football game in the evening, and then he went to a disco with a group of friends. His arm bracelet indicates that he has diabetes. His breath has a fruity odor. His skin is shriveled and dry. It does not "bounce" back when pinched into a fold.

Here are the lab tests of XY's blood:

	patient	normal
Blood glucose	66 mM	4.5 -5.0 mM
pH	7.0	7.4
Ketoacids Acetoacetate and β-OH butyrate	15 mM	2.5 mM
HCO$_3^-$	1.8	25-30 mM
Fatty acids	4.2 mM	0.5 to 2.0 mM
Insulin	Not detected	10-20 units

11.5 Questions regarding diagnosis and treatment of patient XY

What two hormonal sets could cause a coma? When a known diabetic patient is in coma, there must be a differential diagnosis as to the cause of coma. Too much insulin can reduce blood sugar to levels where the brain can no longer function. Too little or no insulin can raise the blood sugar levels to very high levels, stimulate keto-acid production, and result in death. In the case of patient XY, the level of insulin was so low that it could not be detected.

Is the patient in a coma because his brain is not getting enough glucose? No. Glucose transport into the brain does not require insulin. The patient has very high levels of glucose in the blood and in brain.

Is the patient in a coma because the blood pH is low? Low pH will cause coma. Low pH means that the blood has more H^+ ions, i.e. the blood becomes acidic. pH is defined as the negative of the log of H^+ concentration. This means that pH 6 has 10 times higher H^+ concentration than pH 7, and pH 5 has 10 times higher than pH 6 and 100 times higher than pH 7.

The answer to this question is yes. The pH of the patient's blood is dangerously low.

What metabolites cause the low pH? Acetoacetate and β-OH-butyrate originate from carboxy acids. Here is what happens to acetoacetic acid in water:

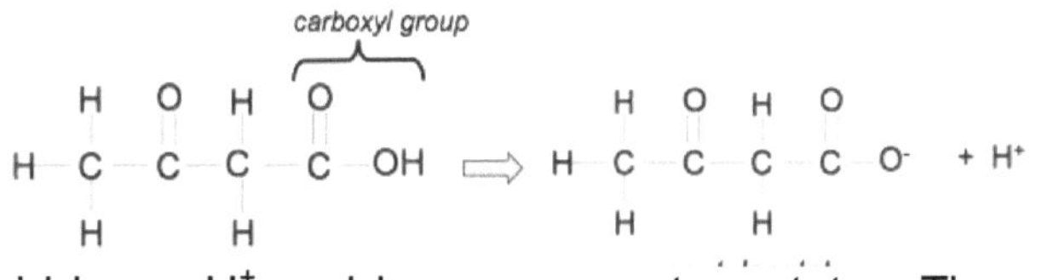

Acetocetic acid loses H^+ and becomes acetoacetate. The same happens with β-OH-butyrate. Both contribute to the increase in the H^+ concentration in the blood and the lower pH.

What pathway or pathways produce bicarbonate (HCO_3)? Pyruvate dehydrogenase and the reactions of the citric acid cycle both produce CO_2. In water CO_2 becomes bicarbonate. The reaction is:

$$CO_2 + H_2O <\text{-}> H_2CO_3 <\text{-}> HCO_3^- + H^+$$

Why is bicarbonate (HCO_3^-) concentration low in the blood of patient XY? When something is low, we always think: "Is it being produced at a lower amount, or is it taken away faster?" In the case of patient XY, CO_2 is being taken away faster than for the control. High H^+ ions force the reaction to go to the left. More CO_2 is lost in the lungs.

Why are fatty acids high? Low insulin stimulates the release of fatty acids from the adipose tissue. The fatty acids are transported in the blood to the liver bound to albumin.

What accounts for the fruity breath of the patient? Ketoacids smell fruity. (Ketoacids are chemically similar to the compounds found in finger nail polish remover, which is how they smell to me). They are being made from fatty acids in liver.

What pathways lead to high ketoacids? First, low insulin and high glucogon causes a breakdown in fat in the adipose tissue. The **fat gets broken** down to fatty acids and glycerol. Fatty acids go into the liver and

119

they get broken to acetyl CoA **by β-oxidation**. Acetyl CoA gets transformed into ketoacids by **ketoacid synthesis pathway.**

How do the levels of ketoacids in the diabetic patient compare with the level of ketoacids in GB during long-term fasting (Chapter 7)? The levels of ketoacids in blood during long-term fasting is about 7 to 8 mM – much lower than in our patient, XY. During fasting, there is still a low level of insulin. The insulin prevents the ketoacids to go to higher levels. The pH of the blood does not drop during long-term fasting.

What does the skin condition tell you about the patient? The patient is dehydrated. Kidney removes some of the glucose from the blood, and the patient's urine will test positive for glucose. In the transport of glucose to the urine, water is also transferred. A patient who has high glucose experiences thirst, but still gets dehydrated because he has frequent urination.

What do you do for treatment? The primary problem is that XY does not have insulin. Insulin is absolutely required for human metabolism. The patient needs to be given insulin. For immediate treatment, the patient's blood has a low pH. Intravenous (IV) infusion of bicarbonate (HCO_3^-) would raise the pH. The patient is also severely dehydrated, and needs fluid in general. As a result of dehydration, the patient's electrolytes (Na, K) in the blood are disturbed. He would have lost Na (sodium) and K (potassium), and if just water were given by IV, the Na and K in his blood plasma would be too low. The physician is especially concerned about the loss of K, since low K can cause heart beating to become irregular.

Now we think about the long-term treatment of the patient

XY carries a syringe of glucogon. He is advised to use it if he ever over-doses with insulin, and his blood glucose drops. Why would a large does of glucogon raise XY's blood sugar? High insulin is a stimulus to store glycogen. Glucogon is the stimulus to break down glycogen to glucose. When the patient is given a pharmacological dose (meaning a dose that is much higher than normally found), then glucogon stimulates the breakdown of glycogen in the liver to form glucose. This glucose goes into the blood stream and raises the blood glucose.

Does muscle glycogen contribute to blood glucose after giving a large does of glucogon? No, for two reasons. Muscle does not have glucose phosphatase, so it can never produce glucose from glucose-6-phosphate. Also, muscle does not have glucogon receptors.

Diabetic patients are advised to keep weight within normal levels. Why would eating excess carbohydrate lead to an increase in cholesterol? Excess carbohydrate is made into fat by the liver. Fat molecules are packaged into a lipoprotein particle, called LDL (low density lipoprotein) that goes into the blood and transports fat to the adipose tissue. This particle requires cholesterol to be intact. The liver makes cholesterol in order to make the LDL particle. Therefore, eating excess carbohydrate leads to increased cholesterol in the blood. Some physicians recommend the use of statins to reduce cholesterol levels in diabetic patients.

12. GB's engine. Recap

We go back to our patient and, by now, our dear friend, Mr. or Ms. Ginger Bread. During metabolism, his body converts carbohydrates, fat and proteins to CO_2 and H_2O, coinciding with making ATP from ADP. At all times, ATP provides energy for nearly everything that occurs in cells.

After GB eats birthday cake, the cake's sugar is transferred from the gastro-intestinal tract to GB's blood. Blood glucose level rises, and the hormone insulin levels rise. Ingested glucose supplies fuel for the brain and other tissues during this phase of eating. Insulin stimulates the removal of glucose from blood, resulting in the conversion of glucose 3 C compounds, pyruvate and lactate, in the cytoplasm by the glycolysis pathway. More ATP is produced when the 3 C compound is converted to a 2 C compound and then to CO_2 and H_2O in the mitochondria (the pathways are pyruvate dehydrogenase, citric acid cycle and oxidative phosphorylation). Insulin also stimulates the storage of glucose as glycogen in muscle and liver. Excess glucose is transformed by the liver to make fat, and fat is stored in the adipose tissue. This removal of glucose from blood allows the blood glucose levels to return to normal levels.

In our story of GB, we noticed that after eating cake, he did not eat for quite a time. Initially, glucose is released to blood from liver glycogen under the influence of the hormone glucogon, and the brain uses this blood glucose for fuel. Muscle also has glycogen, but this glycogen is used for fuel by muscle. Muscle and liver glycogen release from storage are stimulated by the hormone epinephrine. During skateboarding muscle glycogen was broken in the cytoplasm to form lactate and ATP. As GB slowly walked home, lactate in his blood was converted to 2C compound, acetate (in the form of acetyl CoA). Acetyl CoA is converted to CO_2 and H_2O in the muscle mitochondria, concomitant with the formation of ATP.

GB continued not to eat, and he went to sleep without eating. During this time blood glucose is made from amino acids. To make glucose from amino acids requires ATP, and the energy for making ATP comes from metabolizing fat to CO_2 and H_2O in the liver. Indeed, most tissues, except for brain and red blood cells, use fat to make ATP. The heart muscle uses fat at all times. To use fat as a fuel, and to completely oxidize glucose and amino acids to CO_2 and H_2O, O_2 from the atmosphere must be supplied. Within a few minutes of not breathing ATP levels in cells are depleted, and death occurs.

In very long term fasting, fat is made into ketoacids by liver. Most tissues use ketoacids for fuel, however, the liver, which makes ketoacids, does not. Ketoacids are especially important fuel for the brain during starvation. When the brain uses ketoacids it uses less glucose. Since during starvation, glucose is made from the amino acids of proteins, the use of ketoacids spares the breakdown of protein. Since proteins all have functions, the use of less glucose ensures that GB can survive longer. But during starvation some protein continuously breaks down. Eventually, enough protein is lost so muscles can no longer function. With loss of muscle breathing ceases, and with the loss of heart muscle, the heart can no longer pump blood.

Food that GB has eaten, allows him to think great thoughts and do amazing athletic feats. Seamlessly, fuel is used from the diet or from storage, with an intricate cooperation of the organs of his body, working together to utilize food and maintain life.

13. Questions for discussion

13.1 The future?

On every page of this book, there are intriguing unanswered questions that are worthy of further research. Even if you do not become a scientist, it is fun to choose an unanswered question for a "hobby" and then to follow it in the literature over the years. It is surprising to learn the twists and turns that will come out.

Here are some possible areas to follow.

1. **How does well-being affect metabolism and health?** Neurons undoubtedly interact with metabolic pathways. In case of muscle contraction, much is known. A nerve impulse triggers Ca^{++} release from the endoplasmic reticulum. This causes myosin and actin to interact, and ATP to be hydrolyzed to ADP during the muscle contraction. For other pathways, connections between "mind-body" are less well understood. A wise friend told me that development in this important area is hindered because people who know neuro-anatomy do not know metabolism and *vice versa*.

2. **What is the relationship between consciousness and metabolism**? We, and not engines, are conscious. How does memory work? It is known that proteins are synthesized when long-term memories are being stored in the brain. How do we retrieve memories? How do we make conclusions from our memories? The study of brain metabolism is an active field. Brain uses amino acids to make neurotransmitters. The brain is made of a variety of cells, and these cells interact. It appears that astrocytes use glucose to make lactate by glycolysis, and this lactate can be used by neurons.

3. **How is temperature regulated in the body?** Body temperature is very finely regulated, and if the temperature changes by a small amount, the person is sick. How is temperature regulated? What molecules sense temperature in the skin? What sensor in the brain is the temperature regulated?

Some things are known about temperature regulation. There is a special organ that serves to generate fat called brown fat. Brown fat is a tissue that is rich in mitochondria and in fat and this organ is innervated. Babies have a lot of brown fat, and as we age we have less. Brown fat can be seen under the skin of salmon, and the next time you eat a salmon steak you can look for it. (However, please do not gross out your dinner partner by dissecting the fish in the five-star restaurant where you are dining).

If indeed brown fat serves to generate heat, how is temperature sensed? We know how visible light is sensed. A protein molecule, called rhodopsin located in membranes in the retina of the eye, is the light sensor. This molecule contains retinal as a cofactor. Retinal is derived from b-carotene, known as vitamin A, that makes carrots yellow. (Vitamin A can also be found in animal products, such as milk, where the animal has eaten plans containing β-carotene). Retinal has double bonds, and in response to light one of the bonds undergoes a cis to trans conversion (Double bonds and cis/trans configurations of fatty acids were described in Chapter 2). The cis to trans conversion causes a change in the structure of the rhodposin molecule and allows current to go across the membrane. This is the electrical stimulation for the brain to perceive light.

Is something like that happening in heat sensing? Shrimp that live around hot water vents deep in the ocean have a modified rhodopsin molecule in their backs. This molecule absorbs infrared light, i.e. heat, and presumably signals the shrimp when things are getting too hot. Do we have a modified rhodopsin molecule in our skin that allows us to sense heat, i.e. infrared light?

There is a very rare condition when a baby is born who cannot sense heat or pain. This baby does not cry in adverse conditions – not warning the parents when the baby needs help. Consequently, babies born with this condition often have a short life span.

4. What is relationship between genetics and metabolism?

This question is another big one. The sequence of the human genome is largely completed. But at this time, this knowledge does not seem to have produced many practical applications. We know that there are many variants to the proteins in humans. We gave some examples in Chapter 8 in talking about cholesterol, in Chapter 9 in talking about repair of free radicals, and Chapter 10, when talking about hemoglobin. Variants occur in every enzyme in the body, and so every one of us is unique. Will knowledge of a person's unique proteins enable one to tailor diet and medicine for optimal heath for the individual?

5. What is the long-term effect of diet and exercise?

DNA in chromosomes determines the kinds of proteins that our bodies make and proteins regulate all reactions in the body. We inherit DNA from our parents. It was once thought that our DNA from our parents is immutable – what we inherent is what we have. However is now recognized that DNA gets changed during our lifetime. One way it gets changed is by putting a methyl group on it. The study of changes in DNA is a developing "hot" area of research called "epigenetics". These changes are inheritable to the offspring. What causes changes in DNA, how do these changes affect our health, and even the health of our children?

13.2 Questions for review

1. Why do trainers recommend a cool-down period after strenuous exercise? What happens to lactic acid that is in the muscle after strenuous exercise?

During strenuous exercise, not enough O_2 is delivered to the mitochondria to maintain ATP levels through the citric acid cycle and oxidative phosphorylation (Chapter 4). The muscle cells then rely on glycolysis, which does not use O_2. The end product of glycolysis is lactate, an acid. If the athlete uses the same muscles by repeating the same motion, but at a slow rate during a cool-down period after strenuous exercise, enough O_2 is delivered to the muscle's mitochondria to make ATP. Then the muscle converts the lactate back to pyruvate, and pyruvate is removed in the mitochondria (pyruvate dehydrogenase and citric acid cycle in Chapter 4). By this means lactate is removed from muscle. If the athlete suddenly stops vigorous exercise, the lactate gradually leaks from the muscle to blood, but the muscles may feel a bit sore in the meantime. Lactate is taken from blood by liver. Liver can use it to make glucose, or liver can converted lactate to CO_2 and H_2O in the citric acid cycle and oxidative phosphorylation.

2. Why does the brain always need fuel? What fuel does the brain need at most times?

The brain needs fuel constantly to maintain the levels of ions in its cells (K^+ inside and Na^+ outside).

The brain uses glucose as fuel most of the time. The brain uses ketoacids during long-term starvation. (Under some conditions the brain uses amino acids. We did not discuss this).

3. What happens to glucose in the brain?

Glucose gets converted to pyruvate and lactate by glycolysis and then gets converted by the brain to H_2O and CO_2 in the mitochondria using pyruvate dehydrogenase, the citric acid cycle and oxidative phosphorylation.

4. Where does glucose for the brain come from after eating and during short term fast?

The brain uses glucose that is in the blood plasma for fuel. Carbohydrates from eating enter the blood stream from the gastrointestinal tract immediately after eating. After this source is depleted, the liver releases glucose into the blood from its store of glycogen.

5. Where is glucose for the brain obtained during an intermediate term fast? What organ makes glucose under these conditions? Where do the C's for glucose synthesis come from?

Liver makes glucose, using amino acids that mostly come from muscle proteins. The liver releases glucose to blood, and the brain uses this glucose for fuel. To make glucose from amino acids requires ATP. ATP is generated by the conversion of fatty acids to CO_2.

6. During extended fast, what fuel does the brain use?

The brain uses ketoacids in addition to some glucose. The liver makes ketoacids from fat. All tissues except liver and RBC's use ketoacids for fuel. Only the liver makes ketoacids from fat.

7. Many vitamins are cofactors for enzymes.   What are cofactors?

Cofactors are molecules that participate in a enzymatic reaction. They remain within the cell and cycle from one form to another. NAD/NADH, flavin, and ATP/ADP are examples of cofactors. Our bodies make adenosine part of ATP and ADP, so no vitamin is needed. Parts of NAD and flavin are not made in our bodies. We need this from our diet. These molecules are defined as vitamins.

8. Enzymes in what pathways require vitamin B_3 i.e., nicotinic acid? Do you need it every day or every few days? Or can you go for a long time without it?
Nicotinic acid is used to make NADH, NAD, NADP and NADPH. Pathways that break down glucose (glycolysis, pyruvate dehydrogenase and make glucose (gluconeogenesis) require these cofactors.

Nicotinic acid is not stored for a long time in the body. Excess nicotinic acid is lost in the urine. So ideally you should have this vitamin everyday or every few days.

9. Where is the vitamin flavin used in the body? Why do you need it every day or every few days?
Flavin is used in oxidative phosphorylation and the citric acid cycle. It is also used in reactions that detoxify substances. We did not cover these reactions.

Flavin is not stored in the body. It is lost in the urine. We should have this vitamin every day.

10. Where is vitamin B_{12} used? What vitamin is required along with vitamin B_{12}? What groups of people should have supplements of vitamin B_{12}? Can you go for a long time without it?
Vitamin B_{12} is used in the metabolism of some amino acids. It is needed to make lecithin, a major component of membranes. Another vitamin, folic acid, is required along with vitamin B_{12} for 1 C metabolism.

Folic acid is obtained from leafy vegetables. Vitamin B_{12} is obtained from meat and animal products. The animals themselves do not make vitamin B_{12} but obtain it from microorganisms. Vitamin B_{12} is stored in the body, and so a deficiency can take time to develop.

Several groups of people are in danger of developing vitamin B_{12} deficiency. Strict vegetarians, who eschew all animal products, make up one group. People who have stomach or intestinal surgery are another, since both organs are needed for vitamin B_{12} absorption. Finally, the elderly may lose the ability of vitamin B_{12}, and they may become deficient. Since dementia occurs in vitamin B_{12} deficiency, the type of dementia may be misdiagnosed as arising from another age-related dementia.

11. What is "beer belly?" Why does it occur?

Triglyceride, i.e. fat, is stored in specialized tissue called adipose. But fat can accumulate in many cells. When fat accumulates in liver, the liver can become very large, and people call this a "beer belly." A person with a beer belly will sometimes have very thin chest, arms and legs, as most of the body fat has been deposited in the liver.

The interesting question is why does the fat accumulate in the liver. When insulin is low, and glucose is high, triglyceride in the adipose is hydrolyzed to produce fatty acids, which are transported to the liver. If the liver cannot use the fatty acids, then they are reesterified (fatty acids combine with glycerol) to form triglyceride.

12. What disease occurs when insulin is lacking?

Diabetes is a disease that is characterized by high blood sugar. In type I diabetes, the pancreatic beta cells no longer secrete insulin. This causes a raise in blood sugar. In type II diabetes, cells lose their receptors for insulin. Sugar levels rise because insulin is not effective.

13. Which pathways are influenced by insulin?

The pathways that remove glucose from blood, and convert glucose into storage forms are all stimulated by insulin. Insulin affects many processes in the body. Insulin stimulates the transport of glucose into cells, the conversion of glucose to glycogen, the conversion of glucose to lactate and pyruvate in glycolysis, the conversion of acetyl CoA to fatty acids and the storage of fat in adipose tissue.

14. Does muscle use fat during anaerobic exercise?

The oxidation of fatty acid to CO_2 and H_2O requires O_2. If O_2 is depleted in muscle, then glycolysis, using glucose obtained from muscle glycogen, is the source of ATP. Glycolysis does not require O_2. So anaerobic exercise does not directly use fat. However, to restore glycogen after exercise is over, ATP is required. This ATP usually comes from the oxidation of fat. Also, eating carbohydrates after exercise will restore glycogen. These carbohydrates will not be used to make fat, so indirectly, fat stores will be reduced by anaerobic exercise.

15. What is trans-fat? Why might trans-fat be dangerous? An unsaturated fatty acid has one or more bonds in which C bonds doubly to another C. Here is an unsaturated fatty acid:

The position of the two H's bound to the two C's is important. When the H's are on the same side they are said to be in the cis position. When they are on the opposite sides they are called in the trans position. Here is a trans fatty acid:

Most fats in nature are on the cis position.

Fat that enters the body goes into chylomicrons and the chylomicrons circulate throughout the body. The thought is that some of trans fatty acids can be incorporated into membranes. Since, they are not normally found in membranes, some scientists think that they will alter the characteristics of various cell membranes.

16. What is the definition of "organic" in chemistry?

Organic refers to compounds containing carbon. This is one of many words in the English language that have different meanings in different contexts! Fat, carbohydrate and proteins are all considered organic compounds because they all contain C.

17. What is a cation? How do you pronounce "cation?" A molecule has an equal number of protons (positively charged groups) and electrons (negatively charged particles) and it is not charged. An ion is charged; it has either gained or lost an electron. A cation has lost an electron, and then the positive charges are greater than the negative charges. An example is salt, NaCl. NaCl has no charge. But in solution, the Na part has one fewer electron and the Cl has one more electron, and the Na is positively charged; it is a cation. The chloride part has an extra charge and it is negative, an anion.

In chemistry, syllables are strung together without changing the accent. So the root word is ion, pronounced "I on" or "eye on". The addition of cat indicates that the ion is positively charged. Therefore, it is pronounced "cat eye on" not "ca-tion". Anion is pronounced "an eye on". Not really necessary to know the pronunciation, except that you appear more knowledgeable when you use the right pronunciation!

18. What is GM food? Is it dangerous to eat genetically modified (GM) food?
Adding a gene to its DNA alters a food-producing plant. Therefore, the plant makes a protein that the original plant did not. This protein ideally aids in resistance to disease, drought, freezing or another property that would increase the food production or taste of the food. Since proteins are digested to amino acids in the G.I. tract, this additional protein found in the food is unlikely to be harmful to eat. Whether GM foods might be harmful to the environment is another issue.

19. This statement comes from the web: eating denatured protein is dangerous. Is this statement correct? Proteins get broken down to amino acids in the intestine. Denatured proteins will no longer function as enzymes. Consider the green bean. A freshly picked green bean contains mitochondria, the glycolytic pathway enzymes and most of the enzymes that we discussed. It also has enzymes that make chlorophyll and allow for photosynthesis. These enzymes can be isolated, and they can carry out the same reactions in the test tube that they do in the cells of the green bean. When the bean is cooked, the proteins change their shapes, and they are no longer active as enzymes. Once, they are cooked, they stay denatured. Cooked bean tastes different from a raw bean. Another common example of protein denaturation occurs with cooking an egg. Cooking denatures its protein, and once the protein is denatured, it does not become un-cooked.

Cooking, putting the protein in acetic acid (making pickles) or lemon juice (ceviche or pickled herring) are ways to denature proteins of our food. These help preserve food, destroy organisms living in the food, make the food easier to digest and taste better. We humans have been eating denatured food since our ancestors discovered the use of fire. The statement that denatured protein is dangerous is not true.

20. **Another claim from the web: that certain vitamin pills will aid in weight loss. Our question is: will vitamins produce weight loss?** Weight gain occurs when you take in more food than what is converted to CO_2 and H_2O. Many vitamins serve as cofactors for the enzymes used to metabolize food. Table 2, (Appendix), indicates some of these vitamins and reactions in which they are used. In Chapter 4, we indicated that riboflavin and niacin are used in reactions in glycolysis and oxidative phosphorylations – pathways that provide ATP. During dieting, gluconeogenesis occurs. Two vitamins are used as cofactors in pathways that yield the production of glucose from amino acids. Transamination converts alanine to pyruvate (3C), which ultimately is made into glucose. Transamination reactions require pyridoxal or vitamin B_6. Pyruvate undergoes a carboxylation reaction, and enzymes that catalyze carboxylations require biotin. Vitamins that are formulated for "weight loss" usually contain high biotin and pyridoxal. Although these vitamins are needed for gluconeogenesis, the fact is that eating these vitamins will not produce weight loss. Eating less food and exercising more will result in weight reduction.

21. **Some years ago the "alkaline diet" was popular, and it is still used today by a few people. What is an alkaline diet? Do dietary foods have a direct influence on blood pH? Is an alkaline diet beneficial?** Early on, it was recognized that food metabolism in the body and burning produces CO_2 and H_2O. When some food is burned an ash remains. Water added to this ash is alkaline; its pH is above 7. At that time in the late 19th century, it was thought that the components in food that produced the ash helped to raise blood pH.

Look back at Figure 3.1, and instead of a human cell imagine that it is a cell of broccoli. When you eat broccoli, you are eating the whole plant. Outside of the cell, the fluids are high in the ions Ca and K, and inside they are high in Mg and Na. When broccoli is burned, the ions stay in the residue as forms of salt. When water is added to the residue, the water becomes alkaline. In contrast, some of our food is made from storage fuels of plants. For instance, bread is made from flour, which is a plant's storage form of glucose. Oils are plants' storage form of fat. Oil and flour do not have salts. They burn completely to CO_2 and H_2O.

Ion pumps regulate ion levels in cells. Extremes in pH in blood are avoided by HCO_3 (bicarbonate) that forms in blood from CO_2 from metabolism. Eating the so-called "alkaline-rich" foods do not change pH.

Although this diet does not change pH, it may have other benefits. The diet is high in foods where you eat whole cells such as fruits and vegetables. You get vitamins from these foods. On the other hand, the diet is high in K. K is needed for heart function, but too much is bad for the heart. Some people with impaired heart function are advised to avoid high K diets.

22. **Do you get more calories from pyruvate or from alanine?** Pyruvate and alanine are both 3 C carbons. Their pathways of oxidation (Fig. 4.4) yield the same amount of ATP molecules. However, alanine is an amino acid. The N of the amino group must be removed from the body. It gets removed by making urea. It costs ATP to make urea. Therefore, fewer ATP molecules are obtained from alanine.

Appendices

Appendix 1. Name and symbols of elements mentioned in this book

Element	Symbol	Comments
carbon	C	All food contains carbon. Food gets metabolized to CO_2, carbon dioxide
hydrogen	H	H is in all food, and is a part of water, H_2O.
oxygen	O	Oxygen that we breathe is the molecule O_2.
nitrogen	N	Nitrogen is in the amino acids that make up proteins
phosphorous	P	Phosphorous combines with O atoms to make phosphate. Three phosphate groups are in ATP. Phosphate groups are at the surface of membranes, in DNA and bones.
iron	Fe	Fe binds O_2 in hemoglobin; iron compounds are also in mitochondria
sodium	Na	Na^+ is a cation that is mainly outside of cells. Na+ is an electrolyte
chlorine	Cl	Cl^- is a negative electrolyte. It is an anion.
potassium	K	K^+ is an electrolyte that is mainly inside of cells
calcium	Ca	Ca is used for bones and teeth; Ca is needed for muscle contraction
sulfur	S	Sulfur is in some amino acids

Appendix 2. Vitamins, enzyme cofactor, source and deficiency disease

Enzyme cofactor	Enzyme(s)	Source/ deficiency
 Thiamine, vitamin B$_1$	Decarboxylations: Pyruvate dehydrogenase α-ketoglutarate dehydrogense	Whole wheat; beri-beri is disease whe thiamine is deficient (occurs when polished rice is major part of diet)
Riboflavin, Vitamin B$_2$ 	Succinate dehydrogenase (TCA) Fatty acyl dehydrogenase FAD/FADH	Milk, eggs, leafy veggies
 niacin, nicotinic acid	NAD/NADH; NADP/NADPH Many dehydrogenases	Grains, milk, liver Pellagra is deficiency disease (dermatitis, diarrhea, dementia)
 pyridoxal, vitamin B$_6$	Transamination reactions	Wheat, liver meats
 biotin	Carboxylation: pyruvate carboxylase	All foods, liver, milk Deficiency very rare

	1 C	Found in vegetables ("foliage") Deficiency leads to megaloblastic anemia
folic acid		
Vitamin B$_{12}$, cobalamine	Synthesis of methionine from homocysteine. Rearrangement of carbon atoms of methylmalonyl Co to succinyl CoA, making of lecithin, which is a component of membranes	Found in meat. (Animals get it from micro-organisms). Deficiency leads to perncious anemia due to folate methyl trap. Deficiency also leads to degeneration of nerves

About the author

Jane Marie Vanderkooi went to primary school in Amherst, South Dakota and secondary school in Herman, Minnesota. She obtained a B.A. degree from Central College, Pella, Iowa and a Ph.D. degree from St. Louis University in St. Louis, Missouri. She is professor of Biochemistry and Biophysics at the University of Pennsylvania in Philadelphia. She is the coauthor of about 200 peer-reviewed papers.